Praise for *7 Secrets of the Newborn*

"New parents will enjoy this poetic celebration about the love that grows in your heart when you're graced with a new baby. Dr. Hamilton is a gentle and experienced father and physician, and he has filled this sweet book with practical tips and sage insights that inform and delight."   —Harvey Karp, M.D., author of
The Happiest Baby on the Block

"Pediatrician Hamilton offers a cheery, exuberant text intended to celebrate babies, convince readers to have babies, and educate parents about how to best negotiate and enjoy the first twelve months of a child's life. The author, a father of six and grandfather of seven, is clearly enamored by and knowledgeable about his subject. New or prospective parents may very well find his enthusiasm contagious."   —*Publishers Weekly*

"Parents starting out without a big budget or level of experience will breathe a big sigh of relief. The joy of Hamilton's book is helping future and new parents return to that carefree space."
—*Booklist*

"I was an anxious new mother awaiting her interview with pediatrician Robert Hamilton, and Dr. Bob put me at ease, just as he still does today with my now-seven-year-old. Reading his wisdom in this book felt like walking back in time through the first year of my daughter's life. This is the book you didn't know you needed until you needed it."   —Carlie Baiocchi, RNC-OB, ICCE, labor
and delivery nurse and childbirth and parenting
educator at Cedars-Sinai Medical Center, Los Angeles

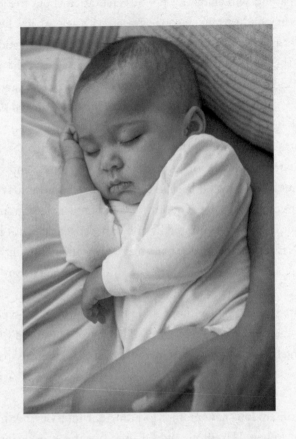

SECRETS AND (HAPPY) SURPRISES

OF THE FIRST YEAR

7
Secrets
of the
Newborn

· · · · · ·

Robert C. Hamilton, M.D.

with Sally Collings

St. Martin's Griffin
New York

Published in the United States by St. Martin's Griffin, an imprint of St. Martin's Publishing Group

7 SECRETS OF THE NEWBORN. Copyright © 2018 by Robert C. Hamilton, M.D. Foreword copyright © 2018 by Patricia Heaton. All rights reserved. Printed in the United States of America. For information, address St. Martin's Publishing Group, 120 Broadway, New York, NY 10271.

www.stmartins.com

Photo on title page by Shutterstock.com
Photo on page 65 courtesy of Ruby Huang, M.D.

The Library of Congress has cataloged the hardcover edition as follows:

Names: Hamilton, Robert C., author.
Title: 7 secrets of the newborn : secrets and (happy) surprises of the first year / Robert C. Hamilton, M.D. with Sally Collings.
Other titles: Seven secrets of the newborn
Description: First Edition. | New York : St. Martin's Press, [2018] | Includes bibliographical references and index.
Identifiers: LCCN 2018022132 | ISBN 9781250114426 (hardcover) | ISBN 9781250114433 (ebook)
Subjects: LCSH: Infants—Care. | Infants—Health and hygiene. | Child rearing.
Classification: LCC HQ774 .H348 2018 | DDC 305.232—dc23
LC record available at https://lccn.loc.gov/2018022132

ISBN 978-1-250-23585-5 (trade paperback)

Our books may be purchased in bulk for promotional, educational, or business use. Please contact your local bookseller or the Macmillan Corporate and Premium Sales Department at 800-221-7945, extension 5442, or by email at MacmillanSpecialMarkets@macmillan.com.

First St. Martin's Griffin Edition: September 2019

10 9 8 7 6 5 4 3 2 1

Dedicated with love to Leslie,

the "wife of my youth"

Contents

Foreword

by Patricia Heaton

If you know anything about Los Angeles, you know it has awful, awful traffic. We do everything we can to avoid getting on the dreaded 405 and the 10 freeways. If you do need to use either of those, there's got to be a very special reason. My special reason was Dr. Bob Hamilton (or, as my son Sam used to call him, "Bopter Dog"). Bob came highly recommended by my ob-gyn, and when it comes to your kids, well, you'll drive the hour-and-fifteen minutes to make sure they are well-taken-care-of.

One of the first things that inspired confidence when my husband, Dave, and I met Dr. Bob was the fact that he had six kids—and he and his darling wife, Leslie, seemed relatively sane nonetheless. So that was encouraging. His office was light and cheery, despite all the crying babies, and his eccentric Harley-riding nurse, Gerri, would pray for your kids right before they got their shots if you asked. Dr. Bob was a very thorough physician. One day he came over to our house and asked to try one of those Razor scooters to see why all his patients were getting hurt. He wobbled down our street for fifteen feet then promptly fell over. Now he knew why.

He knew almost nothing about the entertainment industry as

he didn't watch many TV shows or movies. (I had to constantly remind him how important I am in the real world.) But we had many a lively chat about politics and religion while he was looking in my kids' ears with his auroscope. In fact, when one of my boys was born, Dr. Bob came to the hospital at the same time as my conservative Jewish GP was checking up on me. I would have loved to join in the fascinating discussion that ensued but I was still high on morphine from the C-section. I heard it was scintillating.

Dr. Bob is known for taking incredible care of his patients in Los Angeles. Equally impressive are the trips he organizes multiple times a year to take medical help to developing countries. More than one parent in his practice has joined him on these trips—he badgers us a lot—myself among them. Fifteen years after meeting Dr. Bob, my son Sam (a high school freshman at the time) and I traveled to Sierra Leone along with other doctors and clients. It was memorable not only for the barbed wire and crumbling walls of our "hotel" but also for the incredible amount of organization with which it was run. Dr. Bob has not only brought medical relief to thousands but has also raised funds to build schools and soccer fields. Every year he ropes me into his "Walk for Africa" event to raise money for these trips. His Christianity is not just words in the Bible—he is a true example of faith in action.

Dr. Bob's good works are mostly unknown outside his practice—he's a very humble man. So it was a shock when I looked at my social media and saw a video of him entitled "The Baby Whisperer" with millions of views. The irony was not lost on me. I called him immediately and asked him if he understood what a big deal this was. He didn't really get it (of course). It didn't sink in until he started getting calls from every talk show in New York—some that even I couldn't get on! And what a pro! Dr. Bob looked like he'd been doing TV appearances all his life. I really hoped he would get his own show, or at least become a regular guest on *The Doctors*.

But then again, that would deprive all of us overly anxious SoCal parents of his calming care. So he did the next best thing. He wrote this book.

Dave and I have been so very blessed to have Dr. Bob in our lives. I know that as you read this book, his spirit of joy, hope, and love will touch you. And if you write to him, remind him of how important I am. He still doesn't get it.

Introduction

Human life amazes me!

I have studied biochemistry, human physiology, and medicine for the past forty years. It has been my life's work as a physician, but despite the familiarity of the subject, I continue to find myself utterly amazed by the profound complexity, wisdom, and beauty of the human body. I'm writing this book now for three reasons. First, I hope to bedazzle my readers with the splendor and majesty of human life: both its fragility and yet, at other times, its herculean resilience. I hope my readers will pause for a moment and ponder the curious truth that we are *actually alive and really exist;* that humans are intelligent, conscious, and creative beings who compose melodic symphonies and write novels; that we live and breathe and grow, and somehow, in the midst of the vast chaos of our universe, men and women find one another, fall rapturously in love, and have adorable, *kissable* babies who, like their parents, are *preciously alive.*

My second goal is to convince young people that having a baby is still possible in today's world and that the rewards of parenting are worth all the hassle. I'll admit that being a parent is a challenge, and yes, it requires lots of work, and yes, your children will tax you in ways you never thought possible. Parenting is overwhelming at times. But at the end of the day, child rearing unearths a deeper sense of purpose to every endeavor and renders a fuller understanding of what life is all about. In a sense, children *rescue us* from our pettiness and enlarge our comprehension of reality.

My third and final goal is to celebrate the sheer delight of children. Your infant will bring a smile to your face every day! Few things in life compare to the joy that comes with having a baby, and it would bring me untold pleasure if my readers who don't yet have children would whisper an inconceivable thought that they couldn't imagine they would ever dare utter—namely, "I'd like to have a baby!" Shepherding wary and otherwise distracted young people into embracing the thought of becoming a parent, bringing them to the precipice of decision, and seeing them take the "leap of *yes*" would bring me great satisfaction.

But in prodding young adults to this decision, I must also caution my readers that parenting can be, at times, intensely raw. It is replete with all the challenges that life itself brings. Parenting bruises and stretches us all. But with it also comes a unique opportunity of welcoming a fresh child into the world and watching, from the most intimate perspective possible, a miracle unfold. Women have been giving birth and parents have been raising children for thousands of years. It's still a worthy and doable endeavor . . . and you can do it too!

A Realist with a Flair for the Quixotic

I know how quixotic and retro these ramblings sound. I've articulated some of these musings to friends and family and often get the same response. "Dr. Bob," they say with a smile, "your ideas are quaint and sweet, but you're living in a dream world. You're *so* out of step with what's happening *now* that it's not worth even talking about it!"

Which, I think, is a kind way of saying that I'm insane.

But I'm not. I've just been around long enough to remember a not-so-distant past when the norm for young people was to fall in love, get married, and have children. This was the natural flow of life, and there was little dispute about it.

But I also understand that things are more complicated today than they were when I was a kid. Men and women are building careers. When they complete their educations, good jobs are not always available. College loans come due, and money can be scarce. Life is not as simple as it was portrayed in the rhyming jump-rope ditty that I remember the girls singing during school recesses:

Two little lovebirds
Sitting in a tree
K-I-S-S-I-N-G.
First comes love,
Then comes marriage!
Then comes a baby
In the baby carriage!

To those darling little girls of yesteryear, chorusing in unison to flying ropes on the playground, life wasn't complex. Kissing lovebirds got married and had baby chicks. This was how life was supposed to proceed.

Of course, the rhyme that those jumping girls sang doesn't factor in all the variables of modern life: Does every girl who kisses a boy *really* want to get married to him, much less *have a baby* with him? Did those lovebirds think through their educational goals or their options to travel and see the world?

Yes, those distant-past, jump-rope singers left out a lot, but I still think they got the big picture right, and even though times have changed, their formula still works. Maybe our modern age has made the process of having babies more challenging and expensive, but lovebirds having babies is still a worthy goal, *even today!* All it takes is two people finding each other, falling in love, making a solid commitment to each other, and endeavoring to build a nest together.

The Times Are A-Changin'

Living and practicing in Santa Monica, California, I spend a lot of time interviewing expectant couples. That's because the soon-to-be parents in our community schedule prenatal doctor interviews in advance of their child's delivery to find the "right" doctor for their baby. I love these encounters because they keep me current with what's happening locally regarding pregnancy, babies, and parenting, and they also provide me with a bountiful opportunity to ask expectant young couples lots of questions. I find out what their concerns are and what fears they face, and although prenatal interviews are ostensibly designed to allow these parents-to-be the opportunity to interview me, in truth, I am *also interviewing them.* I don't tell them this, but I am. While they are wondering if I am going to be the right fit for their family, I am also finding out a lot about them, gauging their take on parenthood, and assessing their readiness for the job.

During my career, I have interviewed hundreds of expectant moms and dads, and as a rule, these are happy and delightful encounters. More recently, however, over the past few years, I have begun to sense a different dynamic in these conversations. There's something palpable in the air that I don't remember being there before. The questions that soon-to-be parents ask me today are more pointed and even more desperate. An increasing number of the young couples I interview are looking for guarantees, concrete solutions, and promises. What this tells me is this: young, to-be parents are worried. This anxious undercurrent gives oxygen to worst-case scenarios and nagging what-ifs, which effectively extinguishes the frivolity and lighthearted banter from these otherwise pleasant conversations.

Mind you, all expectant moms and dads have worries. Seeking affirmation that all is going to be okay is normal. Young couples wondering aloud if they are going to be up to the task of parenting is something I expect. In fact, a modicum of angst indicates to me that they are taking their future responsibilities seriously.

But I'm seeing an amplification of these normal concerns. The worries of today's to-be moms and dads are now ratcheted to new heights. I think this reflects the helter-skelter world we all live in. Life today seems to be filled with more uncertainty and insecurity for young parents than what I remember from my own experiences. Life also seems to be coming at us faster and faster. We are barraged with more conflicting information than we can ever possibly sort through or digest. Financially, we're also challenged. More and more families need two incomes just to make ends meet, and on top of it all, the world looks like a more dangerous place to live in, much less bring up children in.

I get all of this. I live in this crucible too. It's normal to use caution in these times, but what I am sensing from many parents today is an *overabundance* of caution, a quest for perfection, and a need for fail-safe plans to mitigate all variables. Newly pregnant couples are approaching parenthood like a college class with homework, final exams, and no wiggle room for error. They're doing everything within their power to get it right so they can *ace* the parenting test. More than anything, they hope to be "perfect" moms and dads, but as we all know, such people don't exist in our world.

Not "Throwin' Away My Shot"

In the Broadway hit *Hamilton* (no relation to the author), Alexander Hamilton proclaims that he's "not throwin' away" his shot. He intends to make sure his "shot" will count because he knows that he's going to have only one chance to get it right. *Hamilton* is set in the 1770s, but this "one chance" concept is also a prevailing theme of our time. "You only live once" sells beer and vacation cruises . . . and when it comes to raising children, the message goes something like this: you only get one shot to be a parent, so don't screw it up! The consensus among millennials is this: *parenting cannot brook error.*

This idea of only having one opportunity to get it right only *amplifies* the anxieties of young parents. The friends and siblings who are watching this frenzied parenting circus from the sidelines are starting to think, *This is crazy making!* These outside observers taking this all in from afar are smart folks. They're looking at the landscape of parenthood and are beginning to perceive that raising children is more of a litany of chores than a celebration; it's another 164 items added on to the to-do list. They see parents striving to get their kids into the *right* kindergarten . . . so they can go to the *right* elementary school . . . so they can make it into the *right* junior high and high schools . . . so they can be chosen by the *right* university, and finally, so they can ultimately land the *right* job. And I am not mentioning worrying about what foods are organic or not and, of course, the future of the planet.

So those without children walk away from the hand-wringing chaos and wonder, *Is this what parenting is all about? If so, count us out! Why would* anyone *want to have a child?* In the abstract, maybe the concept of having children is great, but the reality doesn't look all that enticing. Who's going to get on that leaky ship? Why bother with the hassle, and why would anybody want to buy into that kind of loss of freedom? These are the questions many young people, those who don't yet have children, are asking themselves.

And I don't blame them! It can feel scary out there for parents-to-be!

But here is my first secret of sorts, drawn from many years as a parent and grandparent: no matter what the world looks like today, the delights and the infinite pleasures that children bring to parents' lives are still there to be enjoyed. None of the goodness has diminished, nor is the satisfaction gone. Modern culture is trying to back young people into a corner, but they don't have to go there. My recommendation to young couples is this: take a different road, follow the path less traveled, and dare to live what some people would consider a *counter*cultural life.

Start by piercing through and dismantling the ever-demanding, materialist veil that looms large over our heads. Decide to keep things simple. Parenting is your birthright, so don't let money, keeping pace with others, or the challenges of everyday life fog the way. Make it your goal to hearken to a different voice.

Our Story

The day my wife, Leslie, announced to me that we were going to have a baby was one of the most shocking days of my life. My first thought was, *How did this happen?* My second panicked thought was, *What are we going to do now?*

We were both twenty-one-year-old college students. Most of our colleagues, at least the ones that I knew, were doing their very best *not* to have children. It wasn't considered normal at that time (or now either) for young undergraduates to be having babies. More than one well-meaning friend came up and told me point-blank that Leslie and I were both crazy and assured me, with great authority, that having a child at our age was going to destroy us both, along with any career plans we may have.

But what we discovered was quite the opposite.

Despite the normal anxieties that accompanied Leslie's pregnancy—and contrary to the ominous predictions of some of our acquaintances—we found that becoming a mommy and a daddy to our son Josh was one of the most wonderful things that had ever happened to us.

We were elated to be parents!

Yes, it was life-changing, but Josh wasn't a burden. He was a blessing! In fact, he was the cutest, cleverest, and most developmentally advanced boy ever born. We were smitten, and that never changed.

Financially Challenged

From a financial perspective, Leslie and I were both from modest families, and as college students, we were far from being fiscally flush. In a word, we were *broke* and were getting our educations on a shoelace budget and a small government grant. We didn't have too many other options, so we learned how to negotiate parenthood with the minimum of resources.

Josh was never clothed in the latest fashions, but he was always scrubbed and tidy. Nor did he have an abundance of toys. He played with a wooden box of mismatched, scrap-end blocks that I bought from a local carpentry shop, a couple of soft, spongy balls, and a round, cardboard Quaker Oats barrel. And we also had the great outdoors. We took him on daily walks through the neighborhood, to the local parks, and, in the warmer summer months, to the swimming pool in our apartment complex. Ours was a simple life, but what Josh did have going for him was this: he *owned* two starry-eyed, besotted parents who loved him dearly.

Even today, we remember those days fondly.

There Is No Cosmic Competition

Writing now, I hope to resurrect for today's young couples that breezy, carefree state of mind that we knew after I got over the initial shock of Leslie's pregnancy. We have cherished memories of watching her tummy swelling into a ball, of the laughter and astonishment we shared as our little guy started punching against her tummy, and finally, the overwhelming emotional flood that swept over us the moment Josh was born.

Yes, we did our homework, and yes, we prepared the best we could. We went to Lamaze and Bradley prenatal classes and read the baby books out there at the time, but through it all, we never felt a need to perform, nor did we feel any kind of cosmic competition with other parents. We were going to have a baby, and we were happy.

The End of Delight

So what has happened since Leslie and I were having babies, and why do I sense more anxiety than ever among young parents? Where's the delight that we experienced with her first pregnancy? My hunch is that the carefreeness of expectant parents is being slowly eroded by an impossible litany of absolutes, created by a culture that magnifies fear and demands perfection.

These seeds of anxiety that gnaw on the collective psyches of soon-to-be parents come in small bundles of unsolicited comments and "advice," whispered by coworkers, relatives, and a robust media that pumps out unreal images of parenthood. They're morsels of must-haves that no mom or dad can forget, overbearing "If I were you" tidbits from friends, and finally, the hushed and mysterious "Everyone who has ever had a baby" challenges that come from a media brimming with pictures of celebrities blithely strolling their newborns through Central Park.

Now don't get me wrong—not all this un-asked-for counsel that is coming your way is without merit. It's imperative to buy a safe and convenient car seat. *Before* your baby is born is a great time to purchase life insurance. And yes, it's even good to at least begin *thinking* about saving money for your child's education. But there's no need to attend to all this the moment you find out that you are pregnant. Parenting comes at us one day at a time, and fortunately, things tend to sort themselves out along the way.

But let me help you. There are many things that you *do not need to do* the minute you learn that you are pregnant. You don't *have* to go out and buy a new car. Nor do you need to fill your apartment with lots of baby stuff. You can also rest easy about getting your yet-to-be-born child started on the path to Harvard. And finally, you certainly don't need to call a contractor to start remodeling the house. Babies aren't that big. They don't care about having their own bedrooms, and they won't appreciate a shiny, spick-and-span new bathroom of their own. When they feel the need to poo, they'll do what they need to do wherever they are, which usually happens in the dining room when you're trying to have a quick meal.

My point is this: a lot of things aren't necessary to raise a happy and well-adjusted child. I have traveled far and wide and have seen parents who are raising their children with the barest of resources. And guess what? They're doing a great job. You can too.

My Hard-Knock Education

In this book, I will be sharing with you the things that I have learned as a father of six, a grandfather of seven, and a pediatrician for more than thirty years. I'm going to do my best to distill the things that are true about parenting and the joys that come with having and raising children, and I will share them with you.

Some of what I will pass on to you, I've learned by doing things wrong. Pulling out flash cards for my less-than-one-year-old daughter didn't put her on the road to becoming an early reader. Demanding that *all* my children learn to play the violin, no matter how they felt about it, didn't work out quite so well either. I won't go on, but I promise to make you the beneficiary of my errors.

I've also learned much from the many amazing and engaged parents whose children I have had the honor to care for. These are moms and dads who are devoted to their children and thoroughly invested in being parents. I've learned from dads who teach their children how to catch a ground ball and swim, from moms and dads who pray daily for their children and take them to church faithfully, from other (wild and crazy) parents who have taken their children on grand adventures like visiting all fifty states in *one* extended summer vacation, from moms who climb Kilimanjaro with their teenage daughters, and still others who vacation with their children in remote cabins without televisions or telephones. The number of excellent parents whom I know and have known is vast. They are loving people who have enriched my understanding of what healthy and loving parenting looks like.

What Is True About Parenting

In these pages, I hope to share what is true about parenting. This is a tall order, but I'll do my best because the joys of child raising belong to everyone. The desire to have children is a profound yearning that resides deep within the soul. It's an innate truth that emanates from a natural understanding of the flow of life that we possess from our earliest days. But life's truths can be subtle. They don't muscle their way into our day-by-day lives. They're never found in the thunderclap of cultural consensus, nor are they heard in the violent earthquake of change, nor do they manifest in the furious whirlwind of breathless busyness. Truth resides in a soft and tender whisper. It's the gentle voice that beckons and speaks kindly to our hearts.

I'm writing this book hoping to stir that gentle voice.

Babies Are Good!

Finally, this is a *pro-child* book! Let me tell it to you straight: I want people to have babies. Children are essential for all our tomorrows. Healthy cultures and forward-thinking, positive people look at children as a blessing.

And they are!

Through these pages, I want to bring ideas and thoughts that will demystify the journey, infuse common sense into the process, and, finally, encourage young adults who are waffling on having children to buck up and take the plunge!

What's Ahead for You

My first responsibility in chapter 1 is to let you know that those who are about to have a baby are on the verge of falling desperately in love with a total stranger . . . someone you have never met before. So, mommies and daddies, *beware!* This deep and rapturous love is going to sneak up on you and surprise you.

In chapter 2, we'll take a step back into the workshop of the womb, where, quietly, without fanfare, and unbeknownst to an otherwise busy world, *a big bang–equivalent event* is unfolding. In chapter 3, after we talk about another amazing event called *birth*, we'll walk through the first month of life and do our best to appreciate the astounding developmental changes that occur in four short weeks with your baby.

From there, in chapter 4, I'll recommend that you "live off the grid" and avoid as much of the baby stuff that you may find yourself tempted to buy. In other words, keep it simple. In chapter 5, I'll try to convince you that all a child really needs is *you and your love.* In chapter 6, I'll share with you four cornerstones that make for successful parenting.

In chapter 7, we'll take a roller-coaster, month-by-month tour of what to expect during the first year. Together, we'll stand in awe at the growth and development that occurs in twelve short months. The child you fall in love with at birth will be a distant memory when he or she celebrates turning one year old.

In chapter 8, we'll discuss why establishing healthy patterns like eating and sleeping in the first year yield abundant goodness to you and your baby. In chapter 9, I will make a case for the importance of *mundane living* during baby's first year. All the things that you may think are boring are not the least boring to your child.

In chapter 10, I'll explain to you why babies need both a mom and a dad, and in chapter 11, we'll revel in how much your baby is going to change *you*—the new friends you will have and all the new places your children will bring you.

In chapter 12, I'll make my case for resisting screen time completely for the first year, and in chapter 13, I'll encourage you to keep trekking and traveling, even when your baby is young. I don't want to spoil the surprise, but during the first year, children travel *remarkably well.*

In chapter 14, we'll remind ourselves why family—this new family of yours, as well as the wider family you belong to—is very important when you start having babies. Finally, in chapter 15, I'll encourage my readers to carve out time on a regular basis to rest, something we all need to function efficiently.

Just One

If I can perhaps touch one individual, just one soul, and encourage him or her with my words to venture forward into confident parenting, I'll declare victory. I'm writing for that one. If I happen to bring relief, hope, and clarity to the task of raising children to others also, I will be that much more pleased.

Thoughts from a Different Age

Some of the advice in these pages will sound like it is coming from someone who lived in the foggy, distant past—a grandfather, a great-uncle, or even a voice from some ancient civilization. But it's me, just me. The credentials that I bring to the table are the experiences that I have had as a husband for forty-plus years, as a pediatrician for more than three decades, and as a father and grandfather myself.

As a doctor, I have rendered intimate advice to countless parents and patients. I have seen a lot. I've seen what works and what doesn't work. And much of what I have come to *know* works is considered old-fashioned or even countercultural by some. But this is the retro wisdom that this generation needs to hear.

It can be lonely espousing uncommon and unpopular ideas when everyone else is grooving to a different drummer. I know this because my wife and I were looked upon by others as anomalies when we started having children in our early twenties. But we did it! We raised six great kids, and somehow through it all, we made it!

I'm here now to share some of the secrets we learned along our journey.

1

· · · · ·

The Beginning of It All

Secret #1: You Are About to Fall Desperately in Love

It was one of the oddest prenatal interviews I remember.

On the couch, in my pediatric office, sat an expectant couple who were due to have their first child within the next two months. The smiling mother, Josephine, brimmed with excitement as she shared with me the joy she felt anticipating the birth of their first child.

The father, George, on the other hand, sat on the far end of the couch, away from his wife, looking grumpy. His body language, indifferent attitude, and countenance were the polar opposites of Josephine's.

After I listened to this pregnant woman enthuse about her impending motherhood for a good while, I cautiously turned my attention to George and asked how he felt about becoming a father. His response shocked me. With no shame and without hesitation, he told me that he really wasn't excited at all. In fact, he wondered aloud why he even came to their prenatal interview.

Then he looked at his wife and snarled, "Remember, this was your idea, not mine!"

It was, to say the least, a most uncomfortable moment. Certainly, some men feel exactly the way George did, but rarely do they articulate aloud such candor with a stranger (like me) *and* with their partner present. I did my best to keep my composure and continued to probe his feelings. He wasn't kidding, and throughout our conversation, he never backed down. This "baby scenario" was never a part of his life plan, and as the day approached for Josephine to deliver, he only became more vociferous and, as in the case of our prenatal conversation, borderline belligerent.

I would later learn that George was one of those unique individuals who never minces words. He said exactly what was on his mind, no filters required, as his thoughts came to him. Despite the momentary discomfort that George provoked in me that day, in a funny way, I appreciated his forthright manner. But what George *did not* understand at the time of our conversation was this: he was just two months away from running smack-dab into one of the cutest little baby girls this side of heaven, and this little lady was about to melt his cold, barren heart.

And that's exactly what happened!

From the first moment George cuddled his newborn daughter, Rebecca, he utterly changed. Instantaneously, he morphed into the ultimate poster child for doting fathers. George's "born-again" experience transformed him from an indifferent, low-grade-hostile guy who thought he never wanted to have a baby into his daughter's chief cheerleader, a dad who never missed an appointment in my office, and someone who showered me with endless Rebecca stories, photos, and moment-by-moment updates of her developmental prowess.

George's blossoming into enthusiastic parenthood isn't uncommon. Something wonderful happens to moms and dads when they have a baby. Walls, barriers, and fears that some people don't even know exist come tumbling down as a new center of gravity tugs them and guides them into a different orbit. The things that previously were so important or that they thought they could never do without lose their luster in comparison to this new wonder in their lives.

> *Making the decision to have a child . . . it's momentous. It is to decide forever to have your heart go walking around outside your body.*
>
> —ELIZABETH STONE, TEACHER, AUTHOR, AND JOURNALIST

Parents Are Made to Love, and Hormones Rule

I have parents who daily come to my office and share with me, without any kind of prompting on my behalf, the intense and unexpected love they feel toward their newborn babies. It's an emotion different from anything they have ever known. They speak of these feelings as if they have been possessed by an alien, an outside force, but it comes from deep *within them.*

These feelings that new parents sense are indeed profound, but they are not based in nostalgia or random emotions, nor are they magic. They're a derivative of hidden physiological changes that occur within our human frame.

For moms, these feelings are a result of hormones—those amazing chemical messengers produced by small glands residing in the human brain. Hormones are proteins that, after being secreted in the postpartum mother, race through her bloodstream, alter her physiology, cause *actual physical, structural changes* in her brain, and make the experience of being a mother wonderfully desirable and highly pleasurable.

Prolactin is one of these mommy hormones that is manufactured in the brain's *pituitary gland*. It induces a mother's breast tissues to start milk production after her baby is born. Secondarily, as a bonus side effect, prolactin relaxes a mother and promotes a sense of peace and somnolence when she breastfeeds her baby.

Oxytocin is another of these postpartum hormones that activates several events in the new mother. It too is made in the mother's pituitary gland.

The first action oxytocin has is to trigger the letdown of a mother's milk. When an infant begins to suckle its mother's breast, oxytocin is released. After it is secreted from the brain, it travels to a mother's breast tissues and causes the *ductules* inside to contract and release her stored milk to her baby.

Second, oxytocin causes the enlarged, postdelivery uterus to contract down to its pre-pregnancy size and thereby reduces the uterine blood loss in postpartum mothers. Mothers feel the effect of oxytocin on the uterine muscles as "good" contractions, not unlike the contractions she felt during labor but with much less intensity. These postpartum uterine constrictions, occurring whenever a mother breastfeeds her baby in the early days after delivery, are called *afterpains*, which serve to heal and restore the mother's uterus.

Finally, oxytocin, like prolactin, has antianxiety, relaxing properties that promote a sense of well-being, safety, and security in mothers. The higher the oxytocin levels, the more pleasure a mother senses. As well as being released when her breasts are suckled, oxytocin even surges when a mother lightly strokes her baby, kisses him or holds him to her chest . . . all of which fill a mother—and baby too—with a sense of happiness and contentment.

SURPRISE: Not only does oxytocin play an important role in the postpartum mother, the hormone, sometimes known as "nature's love glue," plays an even stronger role in romantic relationships. Researcher Ruth Feldman from Bar-Ilan University in Israel has found that new lovers (women and men too) have *double* the amount of oxytocin in their blood than pregnant women!

Babies Are Born to Be Loved and to Trust

It goes without saying that human infants are totally helpless when they are born. And like their parents, who are falling desperately in love with them, newborn infants reciprocate by falling impossibly in love with their parents. It's almost as if a baby looks up into the eyes of his mom and dad and whispers, "Let's be partners in this process. I will trust you completely, and we will do this dyad thing together."

Babies are helped in this endeavor by biological forces too. Like their mothers, who are experiencing a flurry of hormonal changes that have caused their breasts to enlarge, their pelvises to relax, and more fat to be stored in their livers, babies are likewise being physiologically prepped for a strong and lasting relationship with their mothers.

Ready and Alert

It begins at birth. Babies are born in a state of heightened alertness, which physicians call the *ready-alert phase*. Birth is clearly a highly stressful experience for a woman, but baby doesn't get a free pass either. For babies, birth represents the most significant physiologic challenge they encounter and which they must overcome after the short 266 days since their conception.

In babies, the stress of delivery induces the release of two more hormones called *adrenaline* and *noradrenaline*, commonly known as the stress or fight-or-flight hormones. With these hormones circulating in the newborn blood, when they're born, babies enter the world on a *true* adrenaline rush.

This hyperalert state lasts for a few hours. With wide-open eyes and dilated pupils, newborn babies stare around the delivery room, look at their mothers, and gaze into the bright overhead lights. I'd love to know what they are thinking during these early minutes after they are born. To me, it appears as if they are wondering what just happened to them and where all these strangers came from.

Like the newborn wildebeest struggling to its feet after being born on the plains of the Serengeti, human newborns, in their own way, look around and struggle to understand and behold the world they have been born into. For them, it's a new universe they heard echoes of while in the womb.

After their delivery, this new world greets them with a sensory jolt; from the noises and chill of the delivery suite, to the touch of a warm blanket, to the soft caress of their mothers, and finally, to the reassuring coos of their astonished fathers.

The Allure of Dilated Eyes

It is well known that humans find dilated eyes to be more attractive than pinpoint pupils. This is one of the reason why dinners by candlelight or with dimmed lights are appealing to couples.

Babies are born with dilated pupils because of the surge of epinephrine and norepinephrine in their bloodstreams. Their dilated pupils enhance their attractiveness to their parents and hasten the all-important process of bonding.

Moms too are in a state of hyperawareness, as every mother who has gone through the ordeal of delivering a baby will testify. When her child is finally placed on her chest, it's one of the most glorious scenes imaginable. For months, she has experienced the curious joy of a little person punching and kicking inside her womb. Finally, after the intensity of labor and delivery, she gets to meet her little swimmer.

I have witnessed this event between newborns and their mommies hundreds of times, and it's the most powerful, touching, and feminine of moments I can think of. It's also the encounter that begins one of the most important relationships an individual will ever know.

Looking for Faces

In addition to being awake and alert, babies are born innately wired to look for faces. Multiple studies have shown that babies, in fact, *crave* faces over all other objects. It is written in our DNA. When babies find their mothers' and fathers' loving and joyous faces, the process of bonding begins.

SURPRISE: Researchers in England using 4-D ultrasound images have shown that *unborn* human fetuses, who are presented with a series of patterns (by harmlessly projecting light through the uterine wall), will prefer to follow the pattern that most conforms to a human face while quickly dismissing other random patterns shown to them.

Coauthor of the report that was published in *Current Biology*, psychologist Vincent Reid of Lancaster University said, "We have shown [that] the fetus can distinguish between different shapes, preferring to track face-like [shapes] over non-face-like shapes."

He went on to say, "This preference has been recognized in [newborn] babies for many decades, but until now exploring fetal vision has not been attempted." ("Womb with a View," *USA Today*, June 8, 2017)

Hearing It All

In addition to being born with eyes wide open, babies are also born with highly developed, exceptional hearing abilities and are thus able to recognize and turn toward unique voices. They attend to and recognize especially the higher-pitched voice of their mothers, which they have heard throughout gestation.

Skin to Skin

Babies are born with a highly mature sense of touch. When the harrowing process of labor and delivery is over, a mother has a desperate desire to hold and touch her baby. As nature would have it, babies are also in need of their mothers' touch and love to be cuddled.

Researchers have demonstrated that frequent and long periods of skin-to-skin contact between mother and child induce a strong bond between them. These studies further show that mothers who have extended skin-to-skin interaction with their babies in the first hours and days of life also end up *breastfeeding* their children for longer periods. The positive benefits of early skin-to-skin contact have been repeatedly confirmed and now has become standard practice in hospitals throughout the United States.

Even in the neonatal intensive care unit (NICU), things are beginning to change. Several hospitals are now remodeling and remaking their neonatal suites to promote "kangaroo care," a treatment plan that allows moms and babies to be with each other and touch one another as much as possible. Research shows that skin-to-skin contact, even with tiny, preterm babies, reduces their stress levels and helps them adapt to life outside the womb more efficiently. In these newly reconstructed units, lights are dimmed and the rooms are designed to be quiet with acoustic ceiling tiles, insulated walls, and silenced monitors. ("The Neonatal ICU Gets a Makeover," *Wall Street Journal,* June 26, 2017)

Bonding

Bonding is the glue that creates an insoluble covenant between mothers, fathers, and their new babies. Researcher Ruth Feldman has written, "Bonding is the central process that supports human adaption [and that] provides a foundation for neurobehavioral maturation." The moments after birth provide the perfect environment for the process of bonding to occur.

For mothers, the preparation for bonding began during pregnancy. Hormones, at work in the mother from the moment of conception, are preparing her physically and mentally for the task she will soon take on. Structural changes—actual physical changes in the brain—are occurring that literally make her into a different person. Pregnancy tinkers with the mother's brain and releases, as writer Adrienne LaFrance puts it, "a flood of hormones [that] help attract a new mother to her baby."

Mothers are further prodded along the bonding road by physiological and maturational events occurring *in her baby,* which also enhance bonding. Visually, newborns are nearsighted, which means they see clearly those things that are close by. Their focal length (the length they can see objects clearly) is between eight and twelve inches. This is the exact distance between a mother's breast and her face. This is not a coincidence. As we have seen earlier, newborns prefer to look at faces more than anything else. The first face that a baby finds after birth and being placed at the breast is the loving face of her mother. Immediately, from the first moments after birth, the bond between baby and mother starts to blossom.

Ready-alert babies, born with eyes open and dilated pupils, find their parents in a surreal and magical moment. It's a collision of lives that is eternal. Moms and dads, who are likewise on epic, hormone-driven emotion highs, succumb to this jubilant occasion and fall insanely and utterly in love with their new baby. Thus hooked, they happily assume the *new role* into which they have been cast: *new parents!*

A note of clarity needs to be offered here. Bonding is one of those surprises in life that occurs on its own schedule. The immediacy of bonding portrayed above isn't fiction. It frequently happens exactly as I have written, but not always. Not every mother or father falls head over heels in love with their baby the moment she is born.

For some new parents, bonding grows over time. Medical emergencies, like unexpected admissions to the NICU, can interrupt a mother's intimacy with her baby during the first minutes and hours of life and cut in on early bonding. Other women experience such discomfort after their deliveries that it is impossible to focus on anyone or anything other than what they so intensely feel. Other women, prescribed pain-relieving medications to soften postpartum pain, also find that the intensity of the early moments with their child is blurred.

But parents are not to worry. These unexpected bumps in the road after birth don't mean that bonding will not occur. The process is simply delayed but is equally intense when it happens.

Talking with Mothers and Fathers

One of the things I like to do as a pediatrician is ask new moms and dads how having a child has affected them. One mother put it this way: "I never thought I could love anyone so completely!" One father told me, "This is the most amazing thing that has ever happened in my life!" Another father smiled and said, "You mean like having the most fun I have ever known?"

Parent-child bonding plays an important role in the continuance of the human species because it is difficult to raise a child to maturity. An unshakable, intense, and solid commitment is required to complete the job. Fortunately, this impulse is locked within our humanness and comes out of nowhere when we need it. For women, bonding is a rich and wonderful facet of their femininity and their maternal biology.

For men, things are more complex. Bonding in men is equally intense, but it's different. My observation about men and babies is this. Most guys—and I am one of these people—didn't spend a lot of time thinking about children when they were young boys, teenagers, or young men. (Sorry, ladies, but we just didn't.) This is an observation I find almost universally true.

But when men become daddies, the lights go on and things change. *Men become awakened to the world of children.* I am a witness to these transformations that occur in men, like our friend George, each day in my office, and this is one of the many reasons I find practicing pediatrics so gratifying.

Preparing for Breastfeeding

Inherent in the early trust a child places in her mommy and daddy is the confidence that she will be protected and cared for.

Breastfeeding is a continuation of what an infant already knows: *a mother's body is the source of all things good!*

From a nutritional and physiological perspective, a mother's breasts replace the mother's placenta. So for a baby to survive, both mommies and babies must adjust to this new outside-the-womb paradigm for nourishment. This means they together need to learn a new skill: breastfeeding.

During pregnancy, a mother's breasts, under the influence of both estrogen and progesterone, are being prepared to nourish her baby. Estrogen and progesterone prompt the breasts to grow fuller and cause the areolae (the pigmented area around the nipples) to enlarge and become darker. Finally, the surrounding oil glands of the areolae (called Montgomery glands) enlarge and mature under their influence.

Estrogen and Progesterone Are Inhibitors of Prolactin

Although prolactin, the hormone responsible for milk production, increases during pregnancy, the high levels of the inhibiting hormones (estrogen and progesterone) prevent milk production from occurring. So while, on one hand, estrogen and progesterone prepare the breasts for action, they also, on the other hand, *prevent* milk production by inhibiting the milk-producing hormone prolactin until the child has been delivered. Since estrogen and progesterone are produced during pregnancy by the placenta, when the placenta detaches from the uterine wall and passes during the final stage of childbirth, the organ that has been producing estrogen and progesterone during pregnancy is gone, and the levels of these placental hormones in the mother's blood plunge.

This exceedingly precise and choreographed hormonal dance then allows prolactin (until now impeded by these inhibiting hormones) to be fully released and stimulate the breasts to start milk production. Once things are turned on and milk production is under way, milk production continues so long as the child suckles and empties the breasts. The more an infant suckles, the more milk is made.

So in review, estrogen and progesterone, which during pregnancy are made *by the placenta*, get the breasts ready for breastfeeding, but also during pregnancy, they *inhibit prolactin*, the hormone responsible for actual milk production. When the placenta is passed after delivery, however, the levels of estrogen and progesterone drop and, thus, prolactin is unleashed from its inhibitors and begins the process of milk production. It all makes sense, and it is all quite wonderful. Milk production *before* the delivery of baby would only complicate matters and make things very, very messy.

Babies Are Ready to Feed

Babies are born ready to fulfill their role in this epic, biological saga too. They're born with an intact and oft-rehearsed suck reflex. Ultrasounds of unborn fetuses show them, as early as twenty weeks of gestation, sucking on anything and everything that they can get their mouths on, including arms, fingers, thumbs, and even umbilical cords! They've been practicing suckling in the womb for half of their fetal existence. Sometimes we see evidence of this when they are born. Large blisters, called *sucking blisters*, are produced in utero by the sucking fetus and are occasionally found on the arms and legs of newborns. They're a testimony to the intensity of the suck of the fetus while in the womb.

So when the big event happens, babies are ready for action and often—just ask any mother; these sweet little newborns become ferocious!

To further the success of breastfeeding, babies are equipped with another reflex. This one literally helps point them in the right direction to find their food. When a newborn's cheek is lightly stroked, the *rooting reflex* causes a newborn to automatically twist his head in the direction of the stroked cheek and open his mouth. A breastfeeding mother, whose nipple lightly touches the cheek of her newborn, happily discovers that her baby willingly turns toward her nipple, opens his mouth, and begins to suckle. It's another small miracle amid an ocean of other miracles, each of which helps to enhance the survival of human babies.

The Beauty of Breastfeeding

A big part of the beauty of breastfeeding is its simplicity. There is no fussing with bottles, no rubber nipples, no formula to prepare, and *nothing to wash!* It's just you, your milk, your love, and your attention, always available, free for the taking, perfectly clean, and delivered at just the right temperature. No other food so perfectly matches what a newborn human being needs.

Colostrum

The first "milk" that a newly delivered mother produces is *not* milk at all but a pre-milk fluid called *colostrum*. It's the antipasto before the main meal. Small in quantity, colostrum is thicker than milk but rich in immunoglobulins, vitamins, and bacteria-fighting white blood cells that protect the newborn from infection. The daily volume of colostrum produced by the mother is about one-tenth the volume of milk that she will make later, but this is all that the newborn infant needs. In addition to supplying nutrition to the newborn, colostrum is also thought to induce the child's immune system to make antibodies and to stimulate the passage of baby's first bowel movement, a black and sticky stool called *meconium*.

SURPRISE: Newborn babies may have a ravenous suck, but they're not all that hungry when they are born. It only looks that way. True hunger will not happen until around three to five days after birth, the exact time a mother's milk fully comes in to quench their need.

As we have seen, breastfeeding also releases the lactation hormones prolactin and oxytocin. As well as playing an important role in milk production (prolactin) and milk letdown (oxytocin), both hormones wash over a mother like a warm shower, inducing a sense of peace and serenity. Breastfeeding is a highly pleasurable experience for most women. It also compels busy moms to stop and spend a quiet and intimate moment with their babies.

How Long Should Moms Breastfeed?

The length of time that moms breastfeed varies greatly, mainly due to cultural norms and the other responsibilities busy mothers carry. As a breastfeeding advocate, I encourage mothers to breastfeed their children for the first year, but I understand that this is difficult for some women to accomplish, especially for those mothers who need to return to the workforce. In that situation, I simply tell mothers I applaud every drop and every day that she can breastfeed her baby. Period!

My recommendation to breastfeed until the first birthday is because, at one year of age, babies can safely begin taking regular cow's milk. So one year makes for a natural transition from breast milk to regular cow's milk for many mothers.

That said, breastfeeding *beyond* one year is perfectly fine too.

Many women will continue to partially breastfeed their children, especially at bedtime and early morning, well beyond the first birthday to maintain a time of intimacy with their babe. And, by the way, if you don't already know this, breastfed babies absolutely *love* to breastfeed! This is one of the major reasons mothers keep at it. Most babies have no intention of weaning and will put up a fuss if a mother tries to do so.

There is even a growing group of women who breastfeed their babies even beyond the second year. I regard this as perfectly fine, but at three years of age, which is a very long time to breastfeed a child by any standard, I tell moms that it's time to close up the factory.

Tip: Lactation and Teeth

It should also be noted that lengthy and frequent breastfeeding after one year of age is associated with higher rates of dental caries. Mothers who choose to breastfeed after their children's baby teeth are in need to employ good oral hygiene to ensure their child's dental health.

The Challenges of Breastfeeding

I have never known a first-time mother who doesn't deal with nipple pain. Soreness occurs during the first days to weeks after delivery as new moms and babies learn this new skill. Breastfeeding is like a dance between a mother and her baby. Early on, before the mother-child dyad get the knack of working together, they spend a lot of time stumbling over each other's feet and falling down. In a short time, however, Mom and baby become pros, and nursing becomes a pleasure rather than a painful ordeal.

Nipple soreness is often due to improper latch, which results in nipple chafing and cracking. Both are intensely painful and can be discouraging to the point that some women throw in the proverbial towel and quit. Breast engorgement and breast infections (which is called *mastitis*) are other woes breastfeeding mothers encounter.

But hang in there! Be patient and don't give up just yet. Find a certified and respected lactation specialist to help you. The value of nursing to you and your baby is well worth the effort. Studies show that babies who are breastfed have improved immunity, less incidence of allergies, and lower rates of obesity.

SURPRISE: Frenectomies Make a Difference for Tongue-Tied Babies

Some babies are born with a condition called *ankyloglossia*. That's a fancy way of saying that your baby is tongue-tied. It happens when the frenulum, the tether that connects the tongue to the bottom of the oral cavity, is short or projects too far forward toward the tip of the tongue. If ankyloglossia exists, it can cause a nursing infant to have an incomplete, shallow latch. What this means for a nursing mother is *intense pain!* Your pediatrician can tell you if your child is tongue-tied, and a simple procedure called a *frenectomy* will correct the problem.

Equally important are the benefits breastfeeding confers to mothers. Moms who breastfeed have lower incidences of breast cancer and lose the weight they gained during pregnancy more rapidly.

But most important, breastfeeding allows mothers and their babies an opportunity to be together, loving each other and bonding ever more fully.

The Wonder of It All

No one can adequately describe the wonder of welcoming a baby into the world. It ranks as one of the true "Wow!" moments life grants to us mere mortals and leaves us all speechless.

Parents of these little people are further blessed because, while attending to their baby and being, as parents are, totally invested and immersed in the process, they are privy to the many other remarkable events that unfold each and every day before their eyes. From their front-row seats, parents see their fresh, newborn little muffins emerge and evolve through their primordial infancy into babbling, walking, blurs-of-activity toddlers. It is a glorious year!

And it's only the beginning of what is in store for moms and dads who have fallen *desperately in love*.

2

. . . . .

It All Begins in the Womb

I know the day I'm going to retire from my pediatric practice. It'll be the morning that I walk into our local hospital, examine a newborn, behold her wispy hair, listen to her heart, look into her bleary eyes, and *not* feel a sense of awe. When I think, *Aw, it's just another kid, no big deal, nothing special*, I'll be done. When I cease to marvel at the miracle of a new life, I know that this will have to be my final day. I'll hang up my stethoscope and move on out into the sunset.

So far, this hasn't happened. I'm still practicing, because with every newborn that I examine, I continue to feel a thrill. A new person has arrived in our world replete with all of life's potential and wonder.

For me, a big part of the excitement of taking care of children is simply the wonder of it all. I have been a pediatrician for more than thirty years, but I haven't yet been able to wrap my head around the idea that the baby who is crying, breastfeeding, pooing, and peeing in front of me *was developing and growing in her mommy's tummy* just the day before!

How can this be?

I have never gotten over the profundity of the process. Human beings begin their lives inside *another* human being. When you stand back and think about it, it's a bit of an insane notion!

I'm not alone in this wonder. I frequently ask new moms, "Can you believe that this child was in your tummy yesterday?" And even though these women have felt bouncing and kicking for months—not to mention the pain and process of delivery—their nonverbal response is always the same: it's a smile and look of wonderment and disbelief.

And dads? When I observe that these babies were in their partners' bellies yesterday, they look at me equally perplexed. Like me, they're incoherent and totally baffled by what just happened to their partners and to them.

My fascination with children—and newborns in particular—began when I was a young boy. My best friend's mother delivered twin boys. When these preterm babies finally came home, I was part of the group who gathered at their home to greet them. That day provided me with one of my first memories of being near newborns and gave me a heretofore unavailable opportunity to study them close at hand. I particularly remember being fascinated with their tiny fingers and delicate fingernails.

As a frequent visitor to their home, I recall staring at them frequently, sometimes for minutes on end (which was a long time for a young boy), scrutinizing the features of their faces, seeing them respond to the sounds in the room, and ultimately watching them mature over the months and years that I was part of their lives. That experience implanted in me an appreciation for newborns that never changed.

So much of what is amazing about newborns—from fertilization to the formation of a mature infant, fully formed with two eyes, two ears, a beating heart, and a functioning brain—occurs inside the womb, before we even lay our eyes on these freshly minted wee ones. So let's take a step back for a moment and review *how* each unique, miraculous human newborn comes into existence. Pregnancy is the biological equivalent of the big bang, but it progresses quietly and ever so elegantly, day by day, without fanfare in the darkness of the womb.

> *For you created my inmost being; you knit me together in my mother's womb. I praise you because I am fearfully and wonderfully made.*
>
> —PSALMS 139:13,14

It Begins in the Womb

The in utero development of human life is one of the most fascinating events that happens in the universe. The 266 days that it takes to construct a new human being in the womb of a woman is an unparalleled feat of nature.

With the advent of high-resolution ultrasound, MRI, and sophisticated microscopes, the mysteries of human fetal development life have now been more fully revealed. The big questions of embryology, however, continue to remain a mystery. Questions like, *how* does the newly formed zygote know *when* to begin the process of cell division, *how* does it tumble its way down the fallopian tube and know *where* to implant itself in the uterus? Finally, where is the instruction manual to direct this cluster of cells to form a new human? These questions still defy explanation. These are the ponderings for theologians and philosophers as much as they continue to puzzle biologists.

There are other questions too. Why do some lucky developing embryo cells get to become neurons, destined to spend their cellular lives struggling with Einstein's tangled theories of relativity or remembering that first goofy smile of your newborn, while others are assigned to become heart cells? And why still other cells are given the nasty job of bumping and clunking along in life as sphincter muscles in the anus?

I also wonder about the *how*. How is it that these primitive *pluripotent cells* (cells that have the potential to form any tissue in the body) know which tissue to become? Where's the choreographer telling these talented cells where to go and what to do?

The answers to some of these questions are magically and mystically tucked into our DNA. All cells of the body (except for red blood cells) have strands of DNA in them that tell the cells what to do. They direct liver cells how to function as liver cells and kidney cells how to be good kidney cells. The glory of human life is that, more often than not, the cells of the body perform their tasks flawlessly. But before the process gets under way, an egg from the mother must be ejected from one of her ovaries.

> *There are only two ways to live your life.*
> *One is as though nothing is a miracle.*
> *The other is as though everything is a miracle.*
>
> —ALBERT EINSTEIN

Ovulation

The process of reproduction begins with ovulation. Nestled in the mother's ovaries, one of the eggs—*eggs that have been present and waiting since her infancy*—must mature and be released. This is yet another complex process that requires precise hormonal timing. It begins in the brain in a structure called the *hypothalamus*, an almond-sized powerhouse that has many functions, including regulating thirst, normalizing the body's temperature, and even controlling sleep.

When it comes to ovulation, the hypothalamus sends a chemical message to the pituitary gland, the "master gland" of the body, and tells it to release two *other* hormone messengers: follicle-stimulating hormone (FSH) and luteinizing hormone (LH). These two molecular ambassadors circulate through the bloodstream and ultimately find the ovaries. The first hormone, FSH, tells the ovaries to make yet *another* hormone (I told you this was complicated!) called estrogen, which will go to the uterus and tell it to get ready for a fresh egg. The second hormone messenger, LH, tells the ovaries to release one their eggs.

Once released from the ovary, our fresh, newly matured egg (or ovum) floats briefly in the mother's peritoneal cavity before slender and seductive, come-hither fimbrial fingers—located at the ends of the fallopian tubes—coax the fresh, just-released, extruded egg into the fallopian tube's opening. Soft peristaltic contractions then push the egg down the tube toward the body of the uterus.

SURPRISE: The Time It Takes

Ovulation (the release of the oocyte, or egg, from the ovary) and fertilization (the fusing of the oocyte and sperm that occurs in the fallopian tube) are separated by only twelve hours. An unfertilized egg dies within twelve to twenty-four hours after ovulation.

Fertilization

One-third of its way down the fallopian tube, the ovum encounters a swarm of chaotically flagellating sperm cells, a small fraction of the millions of sperm cells that were released after intercourse and ejaculation. These are the lucky ones who have squirmed their way through the opening of the mother's cervix, across the uterus, and into the correct fallopian tube to find our virginal egg.

Of the hundreds of sperm candidates that now surround the much larger ovum, only *one* will succeed in penetrating the two outer layers of the egg. To make it through this protective barrier, the head of the sperm releases a digesting enzyme that clears a path through the egg's thick outer barrier to gain entry. In American football terms, the agile halfback sperm carefully following his blocking-tackle enzyme *scores the ultimate Hail Mary touchdown* by making it into the inner-sanctum end zone of the egg.

After the sperm cell muscles its way through the egg's protective layers, the scene is set for egg and sperm to embrace in the epic event called *fertilization*. The coalesced egg and sperm form a *zygote*, and at that very instant, a totally new, unique human being—unlike anyone living now in the world or anyone who has ever lived—has been conceived.

Somewhere in the universe, there's a band playing with fireworks overhead!

SURPRISE: A Bright Burst of Light

Fertility researchers Teresa Woodruff and Tom O'Halloran, a husband-and-wife team from Northwestern University in Chicago, have shown that, at the moment of conception, when the sperm fuses with the ovum, a bright burst of light occurs. This spectacle provides an exclamation point for the formation of new life.

This bright incandescent flash is due to a rapid influx of calcium ions into the fertilized cell, which then induces a brisk *release* of zinc ions from the zygote. Binding to small molecules, this zinc burst results in a fluorescence that can be seen with a microscope. Dr. Woodruff said that "to see the zinc radiate out in a burst [of light] from each human egg was breathtaking" and gave her goose bumps.

In a personal conversation, Dr. Woodruff explained to me that the brighter the burst, the healthier the zygote is. Or in other words, the brighter the flash, the better the chance that this newly formed zygote is going to make it.

The Three Stages of Pregnancy

Fertilization is the green flag that marks the beginning of pregnancy or gestation. Historically, pregnancy has been divided into three periods of equal length called *trimesters*. Since full gestation is approximately nine calendar months (or ten lunar months), each trimester is about three calendar months in length.

These time segments are a useful planning tool for doctors caring for mothers, but scientists, who look closer at the embryology of the unborn child, have refined the stages of gestation into three periods of varying length.

- Stage one is called the **germinal stage,** which lasts for only two weeks.
- Stage two is called the **embryonic stage,** which lasts for six weeks.
- The third and longest stage of pregnancy is the **fetal stage,** which lasts from the eighth week after fertilization until the delivery of the baby.

The Germinal Stage

The germinal stage of pregnancy runs from conception to full implantation of the fertilized egg on the back wall of the uterus. This takes between ten and fourteen days.

A few hours after fertilization, the newly formed zygote undergoes cell division in a process called *cleavage*, which yields two daughter cells. This is the first step in the development of an infinitely complex new human being.

Further division of these daughter cells, over the course of three days, results in a ball of 16 cells, called a *morula*, which then tumbles from the fallopian tube into the body of the uterus. The morula then fills with fluid and further divides to become a structure of 150 cells. At this point, the larger and more mature morula is renamed by scientists as a *blastocyst*. This blastocyst, over the next ten days, is the structure that attaches itself to the back wall of the uterus in the process called *implantation*.

When Do You Know You Are Pregnant?

Amazingly, pregnancy can be detected as early as eight to ten days after conception. The test is based on the presence of human chorionic gonadotropin (or hCG) in the mother's blood (by day eight) or urine (by day ten). hCG is a hormone that stimulates the mother's ovary to produce another hormone called *progesterone*. Progesterone then "talks" to the mother's uterine wall, telling it to get thicker and make ready to receive a fertilized ovum.

THE UTERUS GETS PREPARED

While the fertilized egg is being gently guided through the fallopian tube by the actions of cilia and fallopian tube peristalsis, another remarkable event is likewise occurring on the membranes that line the uterus.

Like hostesses preparing for guests, the lining of the uterus prepares itself for the arrival of the blastocyst. Epithelial cell microvilli, which are tiny projections from the uterine wall, coalesce into flowerlike structures that project from the lining of the uterus in small mounds. These uterine hillocks are called *pinopods* and represent landing sites for the now "sticky" blastocyst to latch on to. They form one week after ovulation and regress within two days. One of these uterine mounds becomes the site that receives the blastocyst and facilitates implantation. If pinopods fail to form and none are present on the uterine lining at the exact time for the searching blastocyst to land on, implantation fails to occur and no baby is formed.

The timing for a new life to form is precise and perfect.

When implantation does successfully happen, however, the first phase of pregnancy is over and the next phase, the embryonic stage, begins.

The Embryonic Stage

The embryonic stage of pregnancy represents the third to eighth weeks after fertilization. This is the time when the cells of the blastocyst, now securely implanted into the back wall of the uterus, come out of their fuzzy huddle, decide which pluripotent cell is going to where, and begin the process scientists call *differentiation*.

By the time the embryonic stage begins, the implanted blastocyst quickly differentiates into a three-layer primitive embryo. These three layers—the *endoderm*, *mesoderm*, and *ectoderm*—are destined to become the various tissues of the body.

Just three weeks after conception, eyes begin to appear on the proto-head of the embryo. Three days after that, the cells that make up the heart begin to coalesce, and by four weeks after fertilization— just twenty-eight short days—a faint heartbeat is present!

At the end of the embryonic stage, six weeks after implantation and eight weeks after conception, this little future baby is now officially called a *human fetus*. In this astonishingly short period, virtually *all the organs and essential structures of a human have been formed.* This newly christened fetus measures one inch in length—a veritable wee, baby inchworm—and now weighs one-thirtieth of an ounce. Eyes and eyelids, fingers and toes, a nose, a mouth, ears, and every organ in its body is present and accounted for—and if you look very, very closely, you can even tell if it's a boy or a girl.

Baby Boy or Baby Girl?

The egg doesn't have any say in whether your baby is a boy or a girl. Eggs only carry X sex chromosomes. So it's the sperm, which carries either X or Y sex chromosomes, that makes the call. If the sperm cell has a female X sex chromosome, the zygote will be XX and the baby will be a girl. If the sperm carries a male Y sex chromosome, the fertilized egg will have XY sex chromosomes and the baby will be a boy.

Fetal Stage of Pregnancy

The third and final period of gestation is the *fetal* stage. By far the longest stage, it lasts from eight weeks postconception to the delivery of the baby. The fetal stage of gestation is all about maturation and is as dramatic and wonder-filled as the germinal and the embryonic stages.

By the end of the third month after conception, the growing fetus is beginning to assume clear human form, with moving arms and legs and a mouth that opens and closes. The face is distinguishable, with forehead, eyelids, nose, and chin.

During this stage, the fetus grows from a one-inch-long fragile wisp, weighing a fraction of an ounce, into a twenty-inch-long sturdy baby weighing an average of seven pounds and who is now ready for *extrauterine* life.

Our Remarkable Brains

The growth of every organ of the body is remarkable, but the growth of the brain is truly astounding and worthy of a brief description. By the sixth month of gestation, nearly all the billions of neurons in the brain have been formed. *At the peak of fetal brain development, over 250,000 new neurons are forming every minute.* This breathless multiplication happens quietly, day in and day out, as our pregnant mother is going about the routines of life, anticipating the third and final trimester of her pregnancy.

SURPRISE: For the most part, neurons are only capable of dividing and making new neurons, a process called neurogenesis, during fetal life. Neurons will *grow in size* until the teen years, but no new neurons are formed after birth. The one exception where neurogenesis does occur is in an area of the brain called the *hippocampus*, the structure of the brain where memory is stored.

After their formation, neurons migrate to various parts of the brain and begin to further differentiate and specialize. When they arrive at their designated spots, they also begin to communicate with other neurons through *synapse* formation. Synapses are the points of communication between neurons, and they continue to develop through childhood.

Shortly before birth and continuing after birth, a rising crescendo of synapses forms. During the first weeks after a child is born, the brain is forming an astronomical one million synapses each second! From a neurological perspective, it appears as if all the neurons in the brain want to communicate with all the other neurons in the brain. This synaptic bloom that begins before birth and continues after birth lasts only for a short time, but it ultimately produces trillions of neuronal interconnections, twice the number of synapses required for healthy brain function.

Out of necessity, this overabundance of synapses will later be pruned: unused neuronal communications wither, while the essential connections—those that are used again and again—are retained and strengthened. Even at this early in life, the principle of "use it or lose it" is at work within the human body.

But synaptic activity is far from over once we are born. Our brains show remarkable levels of plasticity throughout life with different areas of the brain going through the process of maturation at different times.

Comparing Baby's Brain to the Adult Brain

An infant's brain at birth is a quarter the size of an adult brain. The difference in size is due to the number of interconnections (called the white matter) that occur between neurons (called the gray matter). The size of the brain will double in size the first year of life.

From Mommy and Daddy's Perspective

For the mother, the first couple of months of pregnancy can be times of strange cravings, morning sickness, and excessive tiredness. By three months, the top of the growing uterus (called the *fundus*) can be felt at the level of the mother's pubic bone. The recently pregnant mother is now beginning to "show."

By the end of the fourth month after conception, the fetus is six inches in length and weighs between four and seven ounces. The growing fetus is now kicking strongly against the walls of the uterus, and for the first time, a pregnant mom will feel fluttering and evanescent movements, a phenomenon called *quickening*.

At this time, the mother's ob-gyn can feel the top of the uterus midway between the pubic bone and the umbilicus. Now there is no doubt to anyone that she is pregnant.

At the end of the fifth month after fertilization, the parents can clearly see the external genitalia of their baby in a fetal ultrasound and will know if they are expecting a boy or a girl.

By the end of the sixth month after conception—the end of the second traditional trimester—fetuses start to respond to sounds they hear from beyond the womb, and your child begins learning about the world around them, a world that they will soon enter and experience.

Also by the sixth month, the lungs of the fetus begin to mature; however, if a child is prematurely born at this point in gestation, he or she will require extensive respiratory support, but as a general rule, with the advent of modern neonatal intensive care units, your baby is considered *viable*, which means they are capable of living outside the uterus.

By the end of the seventh month of gestation, the fetus weighs about two pounds, and if light is shined into its eyes, the pupils respond. For the next two months, your baby is going to be maturing and storing fat. The average fetus triples its weight during the final two months of pregnancy in preparation for the biggest challenge of its short existence: *birth!*

How Long Is a Full-Term Pregnancy?

Gestation—the time that it takes from conception to delivery—is generally said to be a period of nine months, but it depends on how you count it. The actual time from fertilization to full-term gestation and birth is 266 days, or 8¾ calendar months. If we use a lunar calendar (28-day interval), gestation takes 9½ lunar months from the last menstrual period (or LMP).

Obstetricians today, however, use 40 weeks as being the length of gestation and will relate a mother's progress in terms of weeks of gestation, despite the fact that 266 days divided by 7 days/week is 38 weeks, *not* 40 weeks!

A Day You Will Never Forget

There are days, and then *there are days!* Giving birth as a woman or watching your partner give birth as a man is one of the most surreal and exhilarating experiences of life. It is a *true slam-bang* moment that will be indelibly etched into the memories of mommies and daddies forever.

The process of birth is initiated *by the fetus*. Space begins to get tight in the womb, which causes stress to the child. The resulting hormonal changes in the infant's hypothalamus stimulate the mother's pituitary gland to release cortisol, which, in turn, prompts the mother's uterus to contract. The process begins slowly and with irregular contractions. Over a few hours, however, these uterine contractions become more regular and intense. The time has come to have a baby! It's also time to call the doctor and head for the hospital.

Most couples anticipate and plan for their delivery for months. They attend birth classes and read all the books, but one of the truths of life is *no one* is ever truly ready to be a parent. Despite our efforts, we're not really prepared until it happens. And then another miracle happens. At the exact moment your child is born, *you're ready!* The planning and reading and thinking through the process help, but the delivery experience is what makes it all come together.

Seven Recommendations for a Great Delivery

1. Get some rest before your anticipated delivery date. If you can take time off from work before your delivery, take it. Preparing, resting, and calming yourself before your delivery are keys to a successful delivery.

2. Go light on birth plans. It's normal and understandable to want to have as much control over your labor and delivery as possible. Requests like skin-to-skin time and delaying the application of antibiotics in your baby's eyes are reasonable. No labor and delivery nurse will deny new parents these requests.

But I caution parents that every labor and delivery is unique, and thus, doctors, nurses, and parents cannot be fully anticipate what will be. There are simply too many variables at play. With this in mind, my observation, over the years, has been that birth plans never quite measure up to what ultimately ends up happening. But the nurses and doctors who care for you during your delivery are your advocates. They are pros in delivering babies because they do it every day. They understand the process, and they are *excellent* in caring for laboring mothers and newborn babies. They also understand why you desire and have composed a birth plan, and almost without exception, they will do their best to accommodate and respect your wishes, *but let them do their job and don't let your birth plan interfere with what is best for Mommy and child.*

3. Be kind to the staff. Having a baby is one of the most stressful events young couples will ever experience, and in the midst of the process, it's easy to forget your manners. That said, it's important that couples realize that the people you meet in the labor-and-delivery unit and who are about to assist you in having your baby have helped thousands of other women deliver babies too. They are highly trained professionals, so respect them, show them *your* kindness, and engage their expertise. I mention this because I have seen couples who, amid the drama of delivery, have lost it. *Big time!* This is never a good idea.

To quote Mary Poppins, "A spoonful of sugar helps the medicine go down." It works that way with people too.

4. Fathers, keep a low profile. Giving birth is a deeply feminine event. You are in the delivery suite as a *visitor*. A wise father is one who quietly asks only relevant questions, renders few opinions, and keeps himself generally invisible. Dads, you have two simple jobs in the delivery suite: love and support your partner *and* let the nurses and doctors do their jobs.

Hold your partner's hand, massage her back, respond to her requests, and tell her—quietly—that you love her dearly and respect her eternally. Done!

5. Fathers, take fewer photographs and movies. The delivery of your child is not a Broadway show. And it's hardly the most elegant moment in a woman's life. Childbirth is a basic, unvarnished, and intense human event that often doesn't follow a script. Yes, having photographs of the first moments in your baby's life is important, but I've observed that some dads are so bloody busy snapping pictures that they *miss* the human earthquake that is happening *live and in front of their very eyes!* Later on, they have to rewind the video to see and remember what actually happened at their child's delivery.

Don't let this be your story. If you are forced to make a choice, childbirth is an event to experience, not photograph.

And if you really want to have the event recorded with all the right angles and perfect lighting, *have someone else do the job.*

6. Have your baby in the hospital. There are options when it comes to giving birth, but one of the responsibilities you have as a parent is to optimize the safety of both Mom and baby. Where is the best location to give birth to a baby? Given the experience of the nurses and doctors at your local hospital's labor-and-delivery units and the resources that are there—like real-time fetal monitoring and a readily available operating room—there is virtually no question that having a baby in a hospital is the optimal choice for baby and Mommy.

Maybe the ambiance of a hospital is not what you want, or perhaps you worry about feeling like a number, or possibly you are looking for a totally "natural" childbirth, unhindered by cumbersome protocols. I understand these desires, but when it comes to the delivery of *your* baby, play it safe.

An easy and ideal birth certainly can happen anywhere, but birth complications are common. An umbilical cord can get wrapped around the neck of your child, for example, and thus compromise the oxygen delivery to the baby each time the uterus contracts. Or a mother may experience an excess amount of blood loss after or during a delivery, which may lead to hypovolemia and circulatory collapse. I could go on, but the goal for every delivery is a *healthy* mommy and a *healthy child* who start life out on the right foot.

7. Don't have your baby under water. Water births are a fad. They may be fancied to be more "natural" to some, but they are fraught with serious consequences if everything doesn't go perfectly right. It's natural for babies to take a big breath the second they are born. Make sure they're breathing in air, not the contaminated water their mothers have been laboring in for the past several hours.

Furthermore, it's been recently reported by the Centers for

Disease Control and Prevention that water births are linked to the development of Legionnaires' disease in infants. The *Legionella* bacteria thrives in warm water and can cause severe, life-threatening pneumonia in individuals with immune compromise—like newborn babies—when they are exposed to the bacteria. ("Legionnaires' Outbreaks," *Washington Post*, June 8, 2017)

You Have Your Baby

I have been to hundreds of deliveries, and there is no more sublime scene in life than seeing parents behold their babies for the first time. It's a wonder-filled, utterly joyous, and overwhelmingly rapturous moment. You did it, Mommy and Daddy! You just had your baby!

3

. . . . .

The First Month of Life

Secret #2: For the First Month, Baby Leads the Way—No Schedules, No Programs, Just Baby (It's a Tough Month)

I'll never forget that first drive home from the hospital to our apartment with our son Josh. After rolling my wife, Leslie, in a wheelchair down to our car with Josh in her arms, I put him in the back seat and then helped Leslie climb in before heading for home.

As we were about to leave, however, I remember taking a moment to look around to see if anyone was watching. No one was. All was quiet. We were quite alone, and an odd feeling swept over me. Somehow I sensed that we were doing something *illegal*. Where were all the adults in the world—those professionals at the hospital who *really* knew how to care for children, those people who were surrounding us and monitoring everything just moments before? Didn't they know, didn't they care, or did they even give it a second thought that they had just released a newborn child, *a sweet, young boy*, into the hands of two hopelessly naive, impossibly ignorant, and completely inexperienced twenty-two-year-old novices?

But no one stopped us, so we just drove away.

I'm a Father!

It was during that drive home that I realized, I think *really* for the first time, that I was a *father*. The word pounded in my head. I was a lot of things at that point in my life: a husband, a brother, an uncle, a son, a premedical student—but a father?

The cute little fellow in the infant carrier was coming home to *live with us*, and from this point on, we were going to have to figure out how to care for him. Josh was depending on us to keep him alive.

I took comfort in knowing that Leslie was more knowledgeable about all things parenting than I was and that she was committed to being a great mother. I also appreciated that, from the moment Josh was born, Leslie was madly in love with him and sold on the challenge of mothering. I shared her delight, but my excitement was tempered and mingled with floating feelings of fear and anxiety. What had we gotten ourselves into? I was banking on Leslie's common sense and her motherly love to get us through the first few weeks.

Miraculously, during that first month home with Josh, things worked out. The hours turned into days, and the days stretched into weeks. Every day brought something new. He uttered another sound. He lifted his head an inch higher. He smirked in his sleep. He spent more time awake, started following objects across the room with his eyes, and began to turn his head to voices. Each day was magical. Each day brought more growth and another developmental milestone.

So What *Do* Babies Do During Their First Month?

Pediatricians call the first month after delivery the *neonatal* period. One month is a relatively short span for adults, but for a newborn baby, thirty days represent a full 10 percent of their entire existence, and it is chock-full of remarkable developmental events.

All babies are unique and lovely in their own way, but there are general developmental milestones that new parents can anticipate from their newborns during this month.

Here's my list of what normal newborns do during their first few weeks of their lives:

1. They sleep a lot.
2. They feed all the time.
3. They poo and they pee . . . very frequently.
4. When they are awake, they are constantly moving.
5. Their senses mature.
6. They cry all the time. (And if they don't, consider yourself lucky!)
7. They start mimicking the actions of those caring for them.

1. Newborn Sleep Patterns: After delivery and after their baby's ready-alert phase fades, new parents will notice that their newborn babies *sleep a lot*. The average newborn spends between sixteen to twenty-one hours *a day* sleeping. This inordinate baby hibernation is not, unfortunately, a solid stretch of inactivity. Yes, it's true that the daily *total tally* of time spent sleeping is gigantic, but life is never that easy. Babies' sleeping patterns are broken up into short, two- to three-hour intervals that keep parents busy.

Many newborn babies also haven't yet grasped the concept of night and day. Until their circadian body clocks get on track, they are erratic sleepers who awaken several times during the night and then, conversely, take long naps during the day. This is normal behavior for a baby. Studies show that babies sleep *differently* from the rest of us. They don't spend as much time in deep non-REM sleep as older children, and this is the reason they wake up at the slightest disturbance during the early weeks of life.

There's not much moms and dads can do about their babies' early sleep patterns, and this temporary kink in the road requires an understanding of normal newborn rhythms and a willingness to go with the flow. Of course, this often results in punch-drunk-tired moms and dads who are up several times each night feeding, changing and rocking the baby. Caring for a newborn is a tough job, and when I inquire how moms and dads are feeling at the one-month well-child visit, the word they universally utter is: *exhausted!*

Parenting new babies wears people down, but when I suggest to them, tongue in cheek, that they give their baby to me, I never get any takers. No mother or father has ever said he or she would have it any other way. The joy these little ones bring far exceeds the fatigue and frazzle they create. Moms and dads, after admitting they are tireder than they have ever been, smile the smile of victors and tell me, *despite their weariness*, they have never been happier in their lives!

I call this *good tired*.

Within weeks, however, babies begin to sleep for longer stretches (three to four hours at a time), and they will *naturally* fall into a day/night schedule that eases the burden on parents.

Tip

There's no reason, at this tender age, to begin any kind of rigid sleep scheduling. Formal "sleep training" will come later, but now's the time to allow your newborns to emerge from their postdelivery fog. You can nudge them—for example, turn off the lights and turn down the stereo when it's time for bed—but sleep-wise, let them lead you.

2. **Feeders and Growers:** Newborns routinely lose between 5 and 10 percent of their birth weight within the first four to five days after delivery. This normal and expected weight loss is due to the passage of urine and meconium (newborn black, tarry stools), a newborn's relative indifference to food, and the small quantity of colostrum (a mother's first milk) available.

So when babies get beyond these first couple of days of weight loss, they have some making up to do. When mom's milk *does* come in, around the fourth to fifth day, babies are ready. They enter a period called *cluster feeds*, an avid nursing frenzy, and start gaining between one and two ounces of weight *each day*. Average breastfed babies will recapture their birth weight by seven to ten days after they are born. Most babies go on to gain one to two pounds during the first month of life, and most double their birth weight by four to five months of age.

Like newborn sleep patterns, during the first few weeks of life, you will find that your baby will be highly erratic in her feeding schedule. This is normal, and, like sleep patterns, placing your newborn on any kind of fixed feeding schedule during these early days is unnecessary. Within a short time, however, babies fall naturally into a feeding pattern that is more reasonable. Eventually, perceptive parents can see these subtle changes and nudge their babies along to a more predictable schedule—for example, keeping their baby active and playing to stretch out times between feeding. But for the first month, baby leads the way!

3. **Babies Poo and Pee a Lot!:** Changing diapers is one of the first things young moms and dads learn to master. There's a reason

SURPRISE: Your Babies' Quivering Jaws Doesn't Mean They Are Cold: From time to time, early on, parents also will observe quivering of the lower jaws of their babies. It appears as if their child is chilly, but I assure you, they are not. Like the random movements of their arms and legs, their quivering jaws reflect the immature nature of their neurological system.

for this; it's because new babies are veritable poop and pee machines! So get ready for a deluge.

The first bowel movements that a child produces are black, tar-like, and sticky and are passed within the first twenty-four hours after delivery. These stools are called *meconium* and represent the sloughed cells that first formed the fetal intestinal tract. Several meconium stools are passed over the first few days of life before transitional stools begin.

Transitional bowel movements are looser, green brown in color, and may contain white milk curds. Finally, around one week of life, infants begin passing yellow to green (and sometimes even orange), pasty stools that lack an offensive odor. These are normal breastfed baby bowel movements that young parents will know well.

Babies produce as many as twelve bowel movements per day. That is the outside range of normal, but generally babies normally pass five to eight bowel movements daily.

Oddly, and for no known reason, other young babies will have the complete opposite pattern—namely, *a paucity of bowel movements* during the first months of life. Some will not have a bowel movement for up to *an entire week*. This is also considered to be within the normal range if they don't show discomfort and if the stools, when they *are* passed, are soft and consistent with normal breastfed bowel movements.

Regarding urination, babies also make and pass lots of urine. This is because they are essentially ingesting and living on a liquid diet. Also, young, newborn kidneys do not have the ability to concentrate urine, and thus, they produce and urinate a more dilute urine frequently.

SURPRISE: Guess what, dads? You are about to become amazingly facile in changing diapers! Accept diaper duty as your contribution to the task early child-raising demands. Your willingness to participate in the "duty of doo-doo" is a vital contribution.

4. Babies Get Buff!: It doesn't look like much, but from the minute babies are born, they are working out and getting stronger. In fact, they've already been exercising for the many months that they were floating around inside their mothers' wombs. Just ask any mom about the punishment she endured during her pregnancy and you'll get a vivid account of what it feels like to have an angry and hyperactive gymnast in your tummy. After delivery, they continue their quest to move.

Early on, the movements of their arms and legs are spasmodic and unrefined because newborn babies are neurologically immature. These herky-jerky movements will disappear over a couple of months, and parents will see that their babies' movements will become more deliberate, delicate, and sure.

Tummy Time

Tummy time, even from the very beginning, is likewise important and provides an opportunity for babies to build their core strength. When placed on his stomach, a newborn will briefly lift his chin from the surface of a table and look around . . . before he does a face-plant.

Most babies tire quickly from this exercise and cry within minutes, but the value of tummy time is twofold. First, it helps to strengthen the core muscles of their backs, upper bodies, and necks, and secondly, tummy time helps prevent babies' heads from becoming misshapen, a condition called *plagiocephaly.* Head flattening and asymmetry of the infant's cranium happens when babies are placed *continuously* on their backs. I encourage parents to fit twenty to thirty minutes of total tummy time into each day, broken up into several short sessions.

5. The Five Senses Awaken: Babies are born with remarkably developed senses, and in some aspects, they are more refined and perfected than adults. During their first month, they put their five senses to work.

Their sense of *touch* is highly developed at birth. This is one of the reasons babies enjoy being cuddled, massaged, rocked, and caressed. They naturally nestle with soft and smooth materials but resist scratchy or rough surfaces. They discern the difference between gentle stroking and brisk or rough handling, which makes them cry. Your soft and calm hands convey your love to your baby.

Visually, babies are nearsighted. At birth, they see clearly for a distance of eight to twelve inches, but their visual abilities improve quickly. Within a month, they see clearly to three feet. At birth, they have good peripheral and black-and-white vision, but their color vision is not fully developed until four months of age.

Within the first few weeks of life, babies can track objects that come into their line of vision. They also follow faces across the midline, turn toward lights, and gaze at contrasting black-and-white objects. Moms and dads can enhance their infants' visual awareness with tracking games (moving colorful and interesting objects side to side in front of their infants) and by placing mobiles above the crib for their babies to see.

> **SURPRISE:** Babies have *more* taste buds before they are born than at any other time in their lives.

Taste-wise, babies should be sommeliers. They have *more* taste buds before they are born than at any time of life, and when they are born, they have already been utilizing them to taste (and imprint into their memories) what their mothers have been eating and drinking for months. After birth, they continue to taste what their mothers have been eating in their breast milk. Researchers have found that babies prefer sweet-tasting substances, like their mothers' milk, but their taste buds are not yet sophisticated enough to differentiate between sour and bitter flavors.

The sense of *smell* is also highly developed in newborn babies. Just as they have been tasting flavors, babies have been smelling odors before they were born. Within a few days after birth, babies can detect the scent of their mothers' nipples and even their milk. Researchers have found that newborn babies can smell the difference between their own mothers and other mothers within a few days after delivery. They demonstrate this ability by turning toward their own mothers' breast pads and away from other women's breast pads when given a choice. Inborn instincts lead them to find what they need to survive. Interestingly, this ability to detect a mother's scent is a function of time intimately spent together with the mother.

SURPRISE: Baby Boys and Baby Girls Have Different Sensitivities to Smell

Men and women differ in their smelling abilities. Testosterone diminishes olfactory sensitivity, while estrogen enhances olfaction. This difference is discernable from the very first days of life. Baby girls show more interest in unfamiliar smelling items while newborn baby boys do not.

Bottle-fed babies take longer to discern the difference between their mother's scent and another mother's scent.

Finally, babies also have a highly developed sense of *hearing* at the time of their birth. They heard muffled sounds within the womb from eighteen to twenty weeks of gestation. When they are born, they respond to voices, especially their mothers', from the very start. Studies show that babies tend to respond more readily to higher-pitched voices, which, in part, explains why people naturally (and almost instinctually) alter their voices to a more animated, higher pitch when they interact with babies.

Other studies also show that babies can remember poems and stories that were read to them during their in utero life. Babies whose mothers read aloud the same story or poem over and over during their gestation were found to recognize it when they were born.

6. Fuss and Cry: A full description of the first month would not be complete if fussing and crying were not mentioned. I know there are exceptions to every rule, but for the most part, babies cry a lot! In fact, they cry about everything. If they are hungry, they cry. If they are dirty, they cry. If they are bored, they cry, and if they are tired and want to go to sleep . . . you guessed it, they cry, which is why I affectionately refer to newborns as a bunch of "crybabies"!

Newborn Reflexes

When babies are startled, either by loud noises or a slight drop on their backs, both of their arms will fly out to the sides in a motion that looks as if they are trying to right themselves by reaching out and trying to grab something. This response is called the *Moro reflex*, or *startle reflex,* and it is often accompanied by a shrieking cry. This primitive response goes away within a couple of months.

The Moro reflex is one of several reflexes that newborns are born with, including a *suck* reflex; a *rooting* reflex, which causes them to turn their heads when their cheeks are softly stroked; a *step* reflex, which makes newborns appear as if they are walking when they are suspended over a table; a *crossed-extensor* reflex, which looks like a fencing position; and finally, both plantar and palmar *grasp* reflexes.

And when they are not crying, they're fussing.

The reasons why babies cry and fuss the way they do are not always entirely clear. Pediatricians, however, frequently attribute their irascible ways to gastrointestinal pain and the establishment of the microflora in their digestive tract.

Good bacteria begin growing in the gastrointestinal system from day one and help us digest our food. As babies glide through the birth canal, they are exposed to the normal bacterial flora in their mothers' vaginas and are thoroughly covered with these bacteria. As the birth process progresses, babies end up swallowing these micro-organisms. This natural process provides the "starter culture" for the proper ecology of the baby's bowel microbiota, the bacteria that colonize and make up your baby's gut flora. As authors B. Brett Finlay, Ph.D., and Marie-Claire Arrieta, Ph.D., put it in their book *Let Them Eat Dirt*, "a dirty birth is a good birth."

SURPRISE: There are more "nonhuman" bacterial cells living in and *on* human beings than there are human cells *in* a human.

Bacterial colonization, however, doesn't always go perfectly according to plan. Antibiotics that the mother may have received during or before delivery change their vaginal bacterial milieu. Likewise, antibiotics that an infant may receive in the early days of life may also change the bacterial profile of their guts.

Vaginal "Seeding"

Babies born by caesarean section don't get the benefits of bacterial inoculation from their mothers' vaginal tracts. Therefore, the microbiota established in their guts is quite different from vaginally born infants, and the bacteria that get established in their gastrointestinal tracts is not necessarily the good bacteria that aid in digestion.

To rectify this loss of "good" bacteria, some obstetricians and midwives now swab the newly delivered infant with the vaginal secretions from the delivering mother. Children who have been "seeded" have a gut microbiota that matches that of vaginally delivered infants, which researchers believe protect them from chronic disease, especially allergies.

But even without these extraneous factors, the colonization process seems to be one of fits and starts. Some of the normal bacteria that end up in the gastrointestinal tract are gas-forming organisms. When they get established in your child's gut, they do what they naturally like to do: *make gas,* which parents appreciate as *flatus* almost immediately after the child is born.

In addition to the frequent tooting (which parents like to describe to me in florid detail), these gas-forming bacteria also cause abdominal distention, which frequently causes severe discomfort in infants. Mind you, bloating is a totally *new* experience for the neonate. In the womb, they knew nothing about intestinal distension, and as one may anticipate, they react to their distress with fussiness and crying.

If your baby, however, is exceptionally fussy or irritable or if he has a fever, you should contact your pediatrician.

Ten Things That Make Your Baby Fuss

When your young baby is fussing, the first thing to do is to walk through in your mind the most common reasons:

1. Wet or dirty diapers
2. Abdominal distension
3. Overheating from too many blankets and warm clothes
4. Underdressing/cold
5. Hunger
6. Tiredness
7. Overstimulation
8. Boredom
9. Diapers or clothing that are too tight or uncomfortable
10. Illness

The bottom line is this: when your baby is fussy, walk your way mentally through this list of potential reasons. If things are still unclear and you are unable to calm your baby, it's time to contact your pediatrician.

HOW TO CALM A CRYING BABY

Every mommy, daddy, grandmother, and nanny have their own favorite methods to keep babies content and stop them from screaming. Sometimes nothing works, but there are several techniques caretakers find particularly effective in calming a crying baby.

My friend and colleague Harvey Karp, M.D., has distilled these methods into a system he calls the Five Ss, which he has written about in his book *The Happiest Baby on the Block*. They are:

1. Swaddling
2. Side/stomach position
3. Shushing
4. Swinging
5. Sucking

Any mother or father who has employed any or all five of these simple maneuvers will tell you *they work*. More recently, Dr. Karp has collaborated with others in creating a new, intelligent bassinet that they call the "SNOO." The beauty of this baby bed is it is responsive to the baby. Placed securely swaddled on its back, the baby is calmed by a gentle rocking motion of its head as well as white noise. With the miracle of electronics employed, the bed increases the intensity of rocking and the volume of white noise to match the need of the child. Studies that Dr. Karp has done show that the SNOO helps "mature" a child's circadian sleep pattern as early as two to three months of age.

Incorporating some of the same elements that Dr. Karp delineated in his book, I have devised a technique that I call the "Hold," which is also highly effective in quieting babies during the first two to three months of life.

THE HAMILTON HOLD

One of the tasks pediatricians do when they first meet babies is formally examine them from head to toe to assess their health. We do our physical exams shortly after babies are born and during the subsequent visits to our offices. Almost without exception, when we do our exams, we invariably make these little guys cry . . . and cry like they have never cried before.

So over the years, in an effort to help calm their cries, after finishing my exam, I found myself naturally picking these screaming babies up to quiet them so I could have a meaningful conversation with their parents. That is how my "Hold" was born!

The Hold is a simple technique: the baby is held with her arms

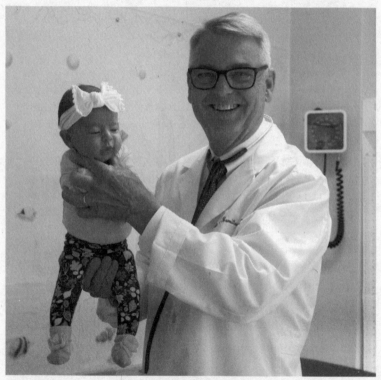

One-month-old Ava in the "Hamilton Hold"

folded one over the other and secured in front of her body with one of my hands. This position inhibits elicitation of the Moro reflex. With my other hand, I hold and secure the baby's bottom.

When I hold the baby *away* from my body and gently bounce her up and down at a forty-five-degree angle, she almost always settles down. If the child doesn't calm quickly, a gentle whisper into her ear or even a finger to suck on works wonders. Although the appearance of this position looks a bit odd to many, it works very well!

As an added bonus, babies who are held in this erect, upright position almost always open their eyes and look around.

A Word About Colic

Colic is a feared word for all new parents. For babies, colic means intense, unrelenting, and prolonged crying for up to three hours, three evenings a week for *three full weeks*.

For parents, colic means miserable evenings and sleepless nights for several weeks . . . and for which there is no simple cure. Studies have shown that giving babies probiotics *can* help, and anti-gas medications (like simethicone) may or may not help. But it's worth a try.

The good news is colic doesn't go on forever and employing either Dr. Karp's "5 S's" or my "Hold" can help calm your child by eliciting the "calming reflex." Around three months of age, symptoms relent and parents get their "old-new" baby back again.

7. Mimicking Babies and Mirror Neurons: During the first weeks of their lives, when babies are awake, they are beginning to look around at the environments that surround them. It's a new world for them: alive, robust, and exciting. They are especially drawn to human faces and begin to mimic them, even from the very start. Andrew Meltzoff, the codirector of the Institute for Learning and Brain Sciences at the University of Washington, has found that young babies have an inborn ability to mimic adult facial expressions and finger movements. This is thought to be due to unique neurons called *mirror neurons.*

SURPRISE: Babies are watching what you do, and they're born to mimic.

Here's how these mirror neurons work. When an infant's hand is stroked, a specific group of neurons located in his brain is stimulated. Now, if this same infant who just had his hand stroked then *sees another* infant having his hand stroked in the same way, the same group of neurons in the observing infant's brain will again light up, *just as if* his own hand was being stroked again.

This was Dr. Meltzoff's amazing discovery. Whether a child is touched or just observing another infant being touched, the same brain activity occurs. This vicarious stimulation represents mirror neurons in action.

Relating this to the social abilities of young babies, Dr. Meltzoff later wrote, "Babies are born socially connected. They see you moving your hand in the hospital room, and they think, 'I have one of those, and I can move it too!'" This innate ability and the yearning of the infant to connect through mimicking the actions of others is present from the start. So within weeks, babies begin mimicking what they see their parents doing. In response to parental goos and coos, they too start cooing and making guttural noises, just like Mom and Dad. *Mind you, this is the cutest thing ever!* New parents delight in their babies responding to them. It's another one of those great "Wow!" moments that moms and dads get to share with their babies.

So, if you want to engage your baby, do what he is doing. If he sticks out his tongue, stick out your tongue. If he yawns, yawn back. In the first month, interacting with your baby is about watching him and letting him watch you. All you need is a comfortable chair, a welcoming lap, and an open heart.

> **SURPRISE:** Your family and friends are dying to meet your new baby.

Friends and Family

There are many people in your life who are excited and happy for you. Throughout your pregnancy, these are the folks who have been encouraging you, helping you prepare, and praying for you. Their delight is genuine, and sharing your newborn with them is important.

In doing so, you will find that your baby will be a great crowd pleaser. Newborn children illuminate every room and bring indescribable joy, especially to your parents, brothers and sisters, aunts and uncles, cousins, and the many, many others who have been championing you through your pregnancy. So open your doors and welcome your friends and family so they can meet the newest addition to the family.

That said, common sense should prevail. Your home cannot become a revolving door or a waystation for relatives and friends. Limits should be instituted as to visiting hours. Dads, this is where you can play an important role. It's critical for mothers to eat and rest properly, have quiet time to nurse and bond with their newborns. Getting into the groove of being a mommy takes time. So,

Daddies, you must become the buffers, the protectors, and the enforcers of your partners' social schedules. Oversocialization, even with well-meaning family and friends, can interrupt the bonding process and interfere with the establishment of early routines for your child.

The first few days after coming home from the hospital can be tough, so I recommend dads establish visiting hours that allow for well-wishers to see both Mom and baby for brief visits. There's no time of the day that is best, but early mornings and mid- to late evenings are usually *not* great times, since these are often the hours when mothers are busy caring for the needs of their babies. Mothers also need to take advantage of their babies' sleeping time to rest as well. Caring for a baby is exhausting work. To recover from the delivery, moms need to take advantage of the moments their babies sleep to rest and sleep as well.

HEALTHY VISITORS ONLY

In the neonatal period—the first month of a child's life—babies' immune systems are untested and immature. They are more susceptible to infections, and not surprisingly, they can get sick quickly, even with simple viral infections like colds. In a baby, this can be a serious business, so parents need to employ prudence when they expose their babies to others.

That said, healthy family and friends are welcome to visit with baby. But the operative word is *healthy*. Dads, this responsibility again falls under your purview. In addition to limiting the number of hours devoted to socialization, you must also concern yourself with the health of your visitors.

It may feel uncomfortable, but it's *not unreasonable* to kindly and graciously ask your various dearly beloved if they are healthy when they call asking to visit your newborn. Some of them will mistake your questioning as rudeness, but hold your ground. I understand that it is awkward to ask your mother-in-law or an excited grandfather if they are healthy enough to visit your baby, so let me give you an out. Blame these obnoxious queries on your pediatrician. Tell your family that your child's doctor prohibits sick folks, even family members, from seeing the baby. People understand this.

The good news is, most people *are* generally healthy and have enough common sense *not* to visit a newborn when they are sick. Young children and toddlers under three to four years of age, however, are the exceptions. These little beasts have virtually no common sense and usually have something dripping from somewhere. So when it comes to having toddlers around your newborn, think twice. In my mind, they're always suspect!

So when your best friend wants to visit your new cherub and bring her three-year-old twin daughters, quiz her thoroughly!

SURPRISE: Early Exposure to Outside/Inside Dogs Reduces the Incidence of Allergies and Asthma Later

In addition to your friends and relatives, your *dog* is also looking forward to meeting your newborn. If you have a pooch, you know that he is keenly aware of what's happening during your pregnancy.

So once you know your doggy feels friendly toward baby (not always the case!), it's okay to let your pup get to know the new member of the family. I recommend that you do so slowly and in a neutral place, like a park. Licks on the face, within reason, are perfectly fine, and many studies show that children who have early exposure to indoor/outdoor dogs have a more varied gut microbiota and tend to have less eczema and asthma later on (*Let Them Eat Dirt* by B. Brett Finlay and Marie-Claire Arrieta, Algonquin Books, 2016, p. 116). As a precaution, make sure your doggy is really healthy and baby-ready. Some doctors recommend taking your dog to the vet before baby comes home.

The Lying-In Period

I was recently asked to do a project with young babies in the People's Republic of China. When I asked my Chinese coworkers to arrange to bring a group of less-than-one-month-old newborns to a hotel for me to examine, they told me that this was not going to be possible. They went on to explain that in China (and throughout Asia), there is a tradition that is rigidly adhered to regarding mothers and children during the first month. It's called *doing the month* (or *zuo yuezi*), and babies and mothers during this time *do not* leave the home except for medical reasons. Strictly enforced by the culture, this custom allows for a time of rest and recovery for both mom and baby—and no American doctor was going to change it.

This time devoted to quietude for newly delivered mothers is not only enforced in China, it is also practiced in many cultures around the world today. It's a unique time that is often surrounded with ritual and tradition. But most important, the postpartum mother is freed from the daily chores of life and enjoys the luxury to collect herself, get to know her baby, and heal in peace.

In Europe and the United States as well, these same cultural restrictions were practiced until the early 1900s. Native Americans call it the *lying-in period*. In colonial America, new mothers were kept in bed for three to four weeks after their deliveries. The women of the mother's family and the community took on all household chores, errands, cooking, and laundry. This period allowed new mothers the time to heal from their deliveries, regain their strength, master breastfeeding, and, most important, bond with their newborns.

The origins of this custom trace back to biblical times. The book of Leviticus mandates a period of purification to be observed after the delivery of a child. If the baby was a boy, the period was for forty days. If the child was a girl, the period was extended to eighty days.

This practice may strike modern Western women as quaint and antiquated, but there is something to be said about giving postpartum mothers a break from everyday responsibilities to recover and rest. While a full month may not sound possible or practical, it's interesting that diverse cultures around the world have all decided on this approximate amount of time for moms to recover.

From my experiences caring for new babies and talking to hundreds of new moms, I can personally verify that one month *is* just about the time that it takes for moms to begin to feel like their old selves again. And for a mother to enjoy an entire month away from all mundane and daily responsibilities, to focus only on herself and her baby, is undoubtedly beneficial for both baby and Mommy.

Cuarentena

In the countries of Latin America, postpartum mothers are kept in the house for forty days in what they call *cuarentena,* or quarantine. During this time, new mothers rest, recuperate, and bond with their babies. As in other cultures, there are rituals that govern this unique time, including binding with a wrap called a *faja* that surrounds the mother's abdomen, as well as special foods to eat and forbidden activities (like sexual relations). Throughout the *cuarentena,* women from the mother's and father's families as well as other women in the community attend to the new mother.

Fresh Air!

As important as it is to lie low during the first month, it is equally important that baby and mom get some fresh air. Even when your baby is young, there is nothing that rejuvenates a new mom more than a short walk around the neighborhood. This, mind you, is a controlled walk in places that are away from crowds. Quiet neighborhoods are great, and parks and beaches are okay too, but avoid restaurants and shopping malls. Enclosed gatherings of people are where viruses get bandied about, and you don't want your less-than-one-month-old infant catching one of them.

After babies are one month of age, I approve a broader exposure to the public. Visits to grocery stores and quiet restaurants are okay, but caution is still to be maintained. By two months of age, after your child has received their first go-round of the important vaccinations, you can become more liberal in your travels and even fly with them. Use caution, however, especially during the winter months. If there is a flu epidemic going around at the time you plan to fly, you may want to reconsider your plans.

SURPRISE: You Are About to Become a Rock Star

Just ask British mother Chelsea Noon what it's like to be a celebrity. She gave birth to a lovely boy named Junior, who happened to have an exceptionally full head of hair. This created a bit of a challenge for Chelsea because Junior became a hometown megastar. So, when she took her "Baby Bear" to the grocery store, instead of getting her shopping done in thirty minutes, Chelsea had to set aside two hours so she could accommodate Junior's many fans.

Like Chelsea, when you have a cute little baby (and every baby is a cute one), the Klieg lights are going to turn on for you. If you have errands to do, take your baby with you only if you have plenty of time. Plan ahead and don't be in a hurry, because people are going to stop you, adore your baby, and want to engage you in conversation.

This is one of the overlooked truths of parenthood. People are simply fascinated by newborns. They will walk across the street or traverse a crowded restaurant to admire them and talk to you.

This rock star status is *particularly* true if you have twins. Parents of twins need to allow even more time (a lot more time) to do even simple errands because they are going to be showered with questions, comments, and salutations every time they go into the public arena. I won't even try to explain what it is like to have triplets.

I regard this in a positive light. People engaging new moms and dads and adoring their babies is a pat on the back to new parents from the community and encourages them in their child-rearing efforts. We are, after all, highly social creatures, and public affirmation of children is one of the more positive interactions new parents come to appreciate.

Babies Are Born with Inner Gyroscopes

Great ships use gyroscopes to maintain their horizontal orientation and keep them stable. Babies also have inner, physiological mechanisms, which, like gyroscopes, monitor every aspect of their inner physiology and keep them stable. This results in a state that scientists call *homeostasis*. These inner monitors tell your baby's lungs how deeply to breathe, her heart how fast to beat, and her kidneys how much to concentrate her urine. And that is only the beginning. Every aspect of your baby's physiology is being carefully and continuously monitored. If things get even remotely awry, her body has the mechanism and ability to keep things in balance.

With this truth in mind, I frequently tell parents an odd-sounding but important piece of information when I see them worrying about caring for their children. "Here's some good news," I tell them. "The baby you are holding *is alive*." They usually look at me a bit confused. I'm not telling them this to be silly but instead to encourage and comfort them. That inner gyroscope, spinning imperceptibly deep inside your baby, quietly leads and guides him on a moment-by-moment basis.

So, Mom and Dad, relax. You do not need to breathe for your baby. Nor do you need to remind him to sleep or eat or poo. They perform all these bodily functions automatically, without any need for assistance. They're well constructed to live on this planet, even during the first month after delivery.

Your job, more than any other, is to be there for your babies. Watch them, listen to them, and adore them. Those early growls, moans, and groans—all those sweet baby noises—need to be heard and assessed.

Amazingly, moms and dads quickly acquire an ability to know their children. Parents soon learn how to crack the crying code. They're programmed with a special kind of sixth sense that allows them, within a very short time, to decipher the peeps and utterances that emanate from their children. They'll know if their babies are crying because they are hungry, in pain, bored, overtired, or even sick. Moms and dads will know their babies.

Young Mothers with Common Sense

Over the past twenty years, I have traveled to Africa and Central America many times, leading medical mission teams to nations that have been ravaged by conflict. While there, we open free clinics and render medical services to children and adults. In caring for the many babies and children in these clinics, I also get the opportunity to interact with their mothers. Over the years, I have met thousands of young—sometimes very young— mothers.

To me, these teen moms look like children themselves. Many of them are illiterate, and almost all of them lack formal education. But despite these apparent disadvantages, the great majority of these young mothers do a *wonderful* job caring for their newborn babies, exhibiting a quality that is hard to teach—namely, common sense—common sense that comes from watching their own mothers and aunties caring for the children in their villages.

These young mothers feed their children when they are hungry, change them when they are dirty, wrap them when they are cold, keep them out of the rain in the winter, and shade them from the sun in the summer.

My point is this: parenting is all consuming, but it's not complicated, and it doesn't require a formal education or special training. But it does require your attention. The first month with your baby is the time to get to know him and study his natural patterns. In a real way, during the first month of life, your baby is going to *teach you* how to be parents. Don't fight it, and resist demanding that your newborn fit into your schedule. That will come later. What is essential is that you listen to, connect with, and concentrate on your baby. The first month is the time to do this.

SURPRISE: Right around the end of the first month of life, your baby starts to smile socially. It melts your heart and charges you up for what lies ahead.

On Our Way to the Orphanage

The first month of life is a prelude to the first year. These first four weeks are when parents get their feet on the ground and begin to develop patterns that will guide them through the months ahead. They are getting to know their little ones.

One of the lovely surprises around the end of that first month is that your baby will look up at you and *smile!* After many tired days and sleepless nights, this is the glimmer that moms and dads so desperately need to keep a steady hand.

I kid that my wife and I were so exhausted by our first son that after the first month with him, we decided to give up and drop him off at the local orphanage. On the way there, however, we chanced to look in the rearview mirror and saw, for the first time ever, a huge, gummy grin beaming back at us. Our bone-weary and stony hearts relented. Throwing up our hands, we turned the car around and headed home.

The first four weeks with your baby are going to knock you flat, so get ready. It's a tough month, but it ends—for you and *your baby*—with big grins.

4

. . . . .

Start Fresh—Live "Off the Grid" and Avoid All the Stuff . . . At Least for the First Month

Secret #3: During the First Month, Your Newborn Doesn't Need Toys, Clothes, a Stroller, or Even a Crib—All Your New Baby Needs Is _You!_

You read that right! I know it sounds preposterous, but for the first month after delivery, you don't need a lot of _stuff_ for your baby. Toys, clothes, cribs, and even strollers are things that get in the way of loving, experiencing, and enjoying your newborn.

During this same short period of time, parents would also do themselves a favor if they put all _their stuff_ aside too. For the first month of your baby's life, things like cell phones and baby apps become distractions.

Think of it like this: the first four weeks with your newborn ought to be a monthlong, skin-to-skin love-in—a super-bonding, thirty-day extravaganza. Do everything in your power to make it so.

The uniqueness of giving birth and the precious and evanescent first days with your newborn are so special, I shudder when I see the experience marred by things—and that includes _anything_ that will compete or interfere with those tender first moments that never come back to you.

There are few times in life like it. Parents need to savor every minute and bask in the sunshine of the treasure they have been given, so my plea is this: don't let material things get in the way.

Toys, clothes, cribs, strollers, and cell phones are all *things*. Turns out, they are wonderful and utilitarian things that, in their proper time and place, are necessary, but if you're not careful, they will interfere with the first-month honeymoon with your baby. As time trickles into weeks and then months, these items will again regain their necessary status, but not now.

A Glut of Gifts

That said, it's hard to keep the avalanche of material things under control. And no matter what your intentions might be and what you do to keep it to a low roar, the plethora of baby items that come your way can be astounding. When you have a baby, your family and friends are going to be very happy for you. As a gesture of their happiness and their generosity, they will want to give you lots of things. That's how people show their love. I regard this as a positive thing, but sometimes, it's too much! Young parents find themselves drowning in gifts, and unfortunately, many of these gifts go unused.

So how is it possible to turn off the deluge without offending those who love you? There's no perfect answer to this "good problem to have," but maybe you can ask a close friend to get the word out to your well-wishing friends and family that your immediate needs have been met, but gift certificates that can be used later to buy diapers and other child-related articles would be appreciated. Gift certificates, of course, are boring. They don't carry the pow and pizzazz that some gift-givers like to create, but in the end, they often prove to be more useful and more appreciated by young parents.

An even more wonderful gift is good, old-fashioned *cash*. Money doesn't make the world go round, but as Jimmy Stewart's character said in the movie *It's a Wonderful Life*, "It comes in real handy down here." Truer words have never been spoken.

Sometimes, for example, finances are not there for parents to take either extended maternity or paternity leaves. This is where a financial gift would make a big difference. Money talk can produce a bit of awkwardness with people, but if you can get over that and if you have family or friends who feel comfortable giving a financial gift that would allow either Mommy or Daddy to stay at home longer with your new baby or address a pending financial obligation, this would be an *invaluable, timely gift* that would be forever treasured.

Six Unbeatable Gifts for a New Mother

There *are* some gifts that are greatly appreciated by a new mother, and I assure you, these gifts *will be* used!

1. Having her partner or a loved one (like her mom) at home with Mommy for the first couple of weeks after delivery.
2. Hiring a mommy's helper to do errands, laundry, household chores, share in some baby care, and cook food for the month.
3. Securing for Mom a comfortable chair in a cozy spot for nursing.
4. Get Mom new slippers and a new nightgown or a new post-maternity outfit—comfy pants or nursing tops.
5. Providing housecleaning for a month.
6. Give Mommy a day at the spa and babysitting to help her get there.

Some Thoughts About Toys

I know families with young children who can no longer sweep their living room floors, they *rake* them. Why? Because they have allowed their homes to become so littered with toys that a simple broom won't do the job. Don't let this happen to you. Don't turn your home into a toy box—and a hazardous place for bare feet—just because you had a baby. And by the way, the majority of these toys will never be played with by your baby in the manner that they were meant to be used. Instead, they are thrown around the room like missiles, employed as hammers to pound on other toys, or simply ignored.

Good toys are objects that bring interest or joy to your baby. For infants, this is usually some sort of colorful article that is soft to touch, safely chewable, and makes noises in response to their touch. As babies grow, good toys engage your child's interest, expand their world, and tickle their imaginations. (See breakout box for a list of true toys for babies.)

> *Your face is your child's first toy.*
>
> —JILL STAMM, *BRIGHT FROM THE START*

Playing with Your Baby

Even from the very moment your babies are born, you can play with them. Playing with babies doesn't require any kind of object, however. It simply involves interacting with them with facial expressions, gestures, and touch.

Author Jill Stamm, in her book *Bright from the Start*, put it well when she wrote, "Your *face* is your child's first toy." Babies are naturally drawn to faces. When offered a choice between faces or other items to look at, from the first moments of life, children always choose faces. Your face is the one thing that they want most to engage, the one object that holds their interest most.

So give your baby her heart's desire: your lovely face. For with your face comes your open and attentive eyes, filled with joy, excitement, and love. And with your face comes smiles, coos, and soft, assuring words that speak to the heart of your newborn baby.

After her first month of life, your newborn will benefit from a handful of simple, cheap, and educational toys like a plush toy to hug, a vivid mobile to follow, and a textured cloth animal to reach out for with her fingers.

But there is no need to fill your house with baby toys, especially toys that are intended for the first month. That said, how many toys does a baby need? The answer is: not as many as you think. Every year, the average family in the United States spends $371 per child on games and toys. In contrast, families in Spain spend an average of $176 per child per year. Three percent of the world's children live in America, but they own 40 percent of the toys consumed globally. The English aren't any better than the Americans. A British study found that the average ten-year-old in England owns 238 toys—but plays with only 12 on a daily basis!

So, if we choose to believe the numbers, we are overwhelming our children with too many toys, toys that they frequently don't appreciate, toys that they don't use, and toys that clog our homes. My recommendation is this: buy toys for your children only after their first month. Find simple toys that fuel their imagination and engage their senses, and above all, avoid toys that *require batteries* to make them work.

True Toys for Baby—After One Month

1. Rattles
2. Unbreakable mirrors
3. Hardback or cloth books with simple, bright pictures
4. Soft, washable, colorful stuffed animals or dolls
5. Small stuffed fabric balls
6. Bath toys

Beware of Batteries

Small batteries are a choking risk for young children. In addition, they can lodge in a child's esophagus or stomach and cause serious mucosal erosions.

No Clothes Either?

Humans need clothing to protect them from the elements. Babies, particularly, have a higher body-surface-area-to-weight ratio than adults and therefore are more likely to become either too cold in cold weather or too warm in hot conditions than adults.

So children do need *some* protection from the environment—but like toys, clothes can also be a distraction. I'm talking about those cute ballerina outfits, the shirts, the jeans, and the frothy dresses, all those outfits that are so delightful for babies to don.

I understand that dressing up your baby can be fun, but when parents are fumbling and futzing with innumerable snaps, zippers, and buttons dressing their just-born babies, their energies are diverted from loving and caressing to an unnecessary task.

By the way, dressing a baby is a challenge for anyone. Little babies are in constant motion. When you push, they pull. What you put in, they take out. And their spiderlike, pencil-thin, but amazingly strong little fingers cling to everything—and they *don't let go.* Just disengaging those fingers from the sleeves of a shirt is a challenge. My point is this: dressing your newborn babies is an effort that requires a lot of your attention—attention that is better directed to loving and cherishing them.

There is another more practical reason why I recommend no fancy clothes for the first month. Your baby is going to plump up and grow a lot faster than you think. Purchasing clothes for newborns is a waste of resources because they are going to grow out of them—you guessed it—in *one* month or maybe even sooner.

So resist the temptation to buy those cute newborn clothes and get your just-born baby a couple of warm blankets, some receiving blankets for swaddling, a sleep sack, and a handful of onesies. Your baby will be just fine, and he will never know the difference. After the first month, you clothes hounds can then go for it. You're free to start dressing him in all the clothes that you got from your friends.

SURPRISE EXCEPTION: Grandmothers and Aunties Get a Pass

I learned early on in my doctoring career not to pick fights with grandmothers and aunties.

I already know that your mother, your mother-in-law, and all your baby's aunties are going to abhor my "no clothes" policy. So here's my consolation. Let 'em have their party, and let 'em dress up your baby to their hearts' content. I know this is fun, and frankly, there is nothing cuter than seeing your newborn daughter in cowgirl duds. Grandmothers and aunties love doing this, so far be it from me to interfere with family traditions.

When It Comes to Baby Clothes, Make Yours a Hand-Me-Down World

Clothes for young babies that have already been used by other children make wonderful hand-me-down gifts. Young infants don't spend much time in the dirt or even on the floor, so their hand-me-down clothes are often in perfect, off-the-shelf condition. Take advantage of this opportunity to save your family some money.

Cribs and Co-Sleeping

When you sleep, your every dream will be filled with thoughts of this new love in your life. So don't put your baby down the hall in another room or even on the other side of your bedroom in a crib that looks like a clunky, wooden cage. Instead, keep them close by your side in a co-sleeper or bassinet.

Cribs will be needed later when it's time to sleep-train your baby, but not in the first month. A simple bassinet (or even the proverbial dresser drawer or cardboard box) next to your bed will do the trick for your newborn baby who undoubtedly will be up frequently at night for feeds and attention.

By definition, *co-sleeping* means sleeping *next* to your infant either by having your baby *share your bed* or *sleeping near* your baby, who is in a separate space (like a bassinet) but within arm's reach. Pediatricians recommend parents *not* to sleep in the same bed as their infants. We *do* recommend, however, that parents sleep next to their babies, especially during the first six months. We refer to children who sleep next to their parents as *near-sleepers*.

There's good evidence that near-sleeping makes good sense. The research on the physiological effects that near-sleeping has on children is, likewise, fascinating. For example, it has been shown that an infant sleeping close to her mother or father will be exposed to the carbon dioxide her parent exhales during sleep. Carbon dioxide acts as a respiratory stimulant for a baby, and thus, this exposure decreases the risk for sudden infant death syndrome (SIDS). Near-sleeping babies also spend more time sleeping on their backs or sides in a ready-to-feed position, which again decreases the risk for SIDS.

Some studies even suggest longer-term benefits of near-sleeping for a child, including less anxiety, higher self-esteem, being more comfortable with affection—even better behavior in school.

No Bed Sharing

Actual bed sharing with newborns is dangerous, especially if smoking, drugs and alcohol, obesity, waterbeds, or couches are any part of the picture. I prefer parents of young babies to use a bassinet or similar sleeper *beside* their beds, but within reaching distance of the mother. Here are the immediate advantages:

- Better sleep—near-sleeping infants startle and cry far less during sleep.
- Stable physiology—babies sleeping beside their parents have more regular temperature, heart rhythm, and breathing.
- Overall decrease in SIDS—in countries where near-sleeping is the norm, SIDS is rare.

Instead of Strollers, Wear Your Baby

Strollers give moms and dads the liberty to get out of the house and into the neighborhood. But they also take young babies *out* of the arms of their parents.

For moms and dads who want to stay close to their babies and get some fresh air during the first month, wearing your lightweight, snuggly newborn in a sling around your chest is the best solution. It's simple, it's easy, and it keeps your baby as close to you as possible.

The advocacy group Babywearing International defines *baby wearing* as "the practice of keeping your baby or toddler close and connected to you as you engage in daily activities [while utilizing] one of a variety of types of baby carriers." While this form of baby transport has been the norm for centuries in many cultures, baby wearing is now growing in popularity in industrialized countries as well.

From ring slings to Mei Tais and woven wraps, there are several low-cost and easy-to-use carriers available that can be utilized to keep your baby close, warm, comfortable, and happy while you carry on with your daily activities.

FOUR BENEFITS OF BABY WEARING FOR PARENTS
Here are some of the reasons why moms and dads all over the world wear their babies.

1. *Hands-free living:* Wearing your baby can make the life of new parents easier. With your baby held tight to your chest, your hands are free to do life's basic tasks.

2. *Getting out of the house made easy:* Compared to toting and folding up strollers, folding up a wrap or soft structure carrier when you're on the go is simple.

3. *Parents feel more confident:* When your baby is right under your nose, it's easier to sense when he is frightened, hungry, or restless, so it's easier to accommodate his needs before his complaints disturb other people around you.

4. *Easier to keep up with older children too:* Parents with older toddlers can keep up with them better outdoors when their new, younger sibling rides along in a sling.

FOUR BENEFITS FOR BABIES

1. *Babies stay content longer:* When babies are worn, they get to enjoy looking at their surroundings and learning about the world around them while having Mommy or Daddy close, feeling their womb-like warmth and hearing their heartbeats.

2. *Increased trust in parents:* When babies know they can easily communicate to their parents when they are hungry, sleepy, wet, or bored, the trust in their parents increases.

3. *Ability to see Mom or Dad's face:* When babies are held close, they can easily see your face. And they love your face!

4. *See and learn from what Mom or Dad is doing:* Babies love to watch their parents. Whether you are preparing food or folding laundry, your baby is watching and learning while seated in a carrier, at eye level with your actions.

Styles of Carriers

- *Ring slings:* Worn over one shoulder with baby in front, ring slings are a popular choice for newborns and infants and can also be used for toddlers.
- *Pouch carriers:* A simple tube of fabric that is worn over one shoulder like the ring sling.
- *Mei Tais:* A modernized version of the traditional Asian-style baby carriers, a Mei Tai is made of one panel of fabric with two long shoulder straps and two shorter straps that go around the waist. While Mei Tais are ideal for older babies and toddlers, they can also be used safely with newborns.
- *Long or short woven wraps:* With a wide variety of fabrics and lengths to choose from, woven wraps are the simplest and most traditional of all carriers. Learning to wrap may seem intimidating at first, but anyone can master and enjoy it with a little practice! Since they have no hardware, woven wraps are great

for snuggling newborns, but they can also be used for toddlers of any age.

- *Soft structure / buckle carriers:* With a thick, padded waistband and shoulder straps, soft structure carriers (SSCs) can easily be worn with baby in front or in back. The straps are adjustable for a custom, comfortable, ergonomic fit, making this the most popular type of baby carrier on the market today.

Before I leave this topic, let me say that strollers are wonderful, marvelously engineered tools that will make your life easier and more doable as your baby grows. But for the first month, keep things simple and save your money. Hold your baby close in your arms and wrap her snugly to your chest.

Mobile Phones Take You Away from Your Baby

Mobile phones are one of the most astounding inventions of our modern world. As a pediatrician, I live on my cell phone, and with the never-ending number of apps available, my cell phone has become the most useful tool I own.

In a word, like a lot of other people I know, I am irredeemably *addicted* to it. I know this because I once lost this trusted friend, and the confusion and total bewilderment that I felt for days after the loss underlined my dependence on it.

When we go to a concert or a movie, however, the audience is reminded to turn off their phones before the music begins. There is nothing more irritating to a conductor or fellow viewers than to have cell phones sound off like roosters in the middle of a musical piece.

Cell phone use during the first month of a child's life also needs to be conquered. Like a musical performance that shan't be interrupted, the first days of your baby's life are sacred, and cell phones represent a disrupting distraction.

So say goodbye to your wonderful electronic friend for a month after your baby is born. Put it on the shelf and let it rest.

Don't lose it, but don't use it either.

Apps Have Gotta Go Too!

Along with your phone, you've also got to park all your apps. There is an amazing array of baby apps that have parents documenting the number of feedings, the frequency and quality of every stool, daily weights and sleep patterns of a child . . . all on a moment-to-moment basis.

Of course, these apps are cool, but they aren't needed in the least. Moms and dads who forgo this blow-by-blow record keeping—whether they use an app or whether they write it down—are going to save themselves hours of logging data that, in the big picture, *have almost zero value.*

When your pediatrician asks you about your baby's daily habits, she is not expecting a computer-generated spreadsheet, nor is she looking for a robust dissertation about every poo and pee your child has ever passed. She's looking for generalities. If you child is not urinating, this is a problem, and you will know it. If your baby has not passed stool for the past week, you won't need an app to answer the question. You will know, and you will be able to give an excellent answer to all your pediatrician's queries. So save your time for more productive tasks, like kissing your baby's toes.

New Parents Only Want the Best

I know that young parents want to do the "right" thing by their children more than anything else. All dads and moms want to get off on the right foot and to provide their babies with the best opportunities they can, right from the beginning. Achieving these goals and knowing what *really* is best for their babies, however, is often confusing in our consumer-based, media-saturated culture.

That said, leveraging this natural desire parents have to do the best they can for their children translates into selling opportunities for those who have products to market. I have nothing against people selling things, but when it comes to babies, most of these things that companies tell parents they *have to have* are unnecessary, especially during the first month. Too much stuff during the first weeks of life only gets in the way of what is important.

So don't go there. Save yourself loads of cash and become a minimalist. Get the basic items you need and no more.

Ten Things Your Baby Doesn't Need

As a new parent, you will be inundated with suggestions on what to buy. Much of it is not necessary at all!

1. Changing table—diapers are most often changed on the fly: in the bedroom, the living room or the local park. Buy a simple waterproof pad that you can put down where and when you need it, or choose a changing table that incorporates a set of drawers or shelves for storage if that is something you need.
2. Baby baths—a large washing-up bowl will do the trick, or even the kitchen sink or even a bucket!
3. Diaper disposal system—most parents want to get used diapers out of the house just as fast as possible, so a pack of diaper sacks and the household trash can solve all your problems.
4. High chair—not only do they take up room, they quickly become encrusted with all kind of food matter. Instead, find a booster-style seat that attaches to a regular chair. Choose the simplest design with the fewest nooks and crannies for food to lodge in.

5. Changing bag—those specially branded diaper bags come with a high price tag. A simple tote bag does the job just as well.

6. Crib—I recommend a bassinet beside the bed for the first six months. After that, a crib that can later be transformed into a bed will last longer and ease the transition to a real bed.

7. Pram, or the traditional baby buggy—this is only useful for the first few months, and then it ceases to have any value at all. I recommend carrying your baby in a sling during those early days. So skip the pram and buy a stroller when you need it.

8. Nursing chair—yes, you need a comfortable chair with good back support for feeding baby, but it doesn't need to be a specially designed furniture item.

9. Playpen—another cage-like device that you don't really need. Babies should explore; just make sure your home is child-safe.

10. Baby food processor—once your baby is ready for solids, steaming and mashing vegetables and fruit doesn't require specialized equipment. All it takes is a fork and a strong arm.

What Babies Really Want

I am not making these "anti" recommendations just to be contrary. Instead, I am giving young parents the liberty to say no to the distractions, to save a bundle of dough, and, as a bonus, to free them to cocoon themselves away from our gadget-strewn world for the first month with their babies.

Toys, clothes, strollers, cribs, and yes, even cell phones are just some of the more obvious distractions that divert parents' attention from their babies. There are many others. But for one month—one very short month—I hope moms and dads will step back and do nothing else but relish their babies. That they will value those ephemeral moments to enjoy, appreciate, and bond with the new love of their lives in the most intimate, deep, and *quiet* way they can, unencumbered by the whirl and whiz of material stuff.

Each minute of your baby's fresh new life is infinitely precious, and once they slip past, we never get them back. Treasure the riches of each day, and do not commit the common error of getting lost with *things*.

I am also making these recommendations as an advocate for your baby. What they need and what they want more than anything is *you!*

You without any competition. You without distractions. You without the muddle of extraneous stuff. Just you.

Off-the-Grid Living

Finally, in recommending that parents go without lots of stuff and live an off-the-grid existence for the first month after your baby is born, I'm hoping that some of this simple lifestyle sticks. If you can adjust to leaner living—not only for the first month but for the months and years ahead—you and your family will enjoy deeper and fuller lives. Acquiring and having things has never satisfied the souls of human beings anyway. We know this in our hearts, but the temptation to *have things* is almost impossible to overcome, especially if we deem these things to be of value to our children. We all want the best for our children, but the "best" for them is usually not more stuff.

I am far from a neo-bohemian, nor do I advocate returning to hippie life. I once lived on a commune and know firsthand the shortcomings of "back to the earth" idealism. I also know that I am unlikely to single-handedly push back the materialism and hyperconsumerism that has infected our world. And really, I am not interested in engaging that battle. I'll leave that to the preachers and others to sort out. I know the nature of human beings. We are jealous creatures who envy what others possess and want what others have.

But there *are elements* of the monastic, simpler, Walden Pond lifestyle that are meritorious. And maybe some readers who take my minimalistic "no toys, no clothes, no strollers, no cribs, and no cell phones" prescription for the first month of their babies' lives will come out on the other side of that first month and keep going. To some, minimalism may sound unpleasant or even impossible, but it is eminently doable. So, new dads and moms, you have permission to live a simpler and *easier* life, free from chaos and clutter and full of familial love and meaningful interactions.

In the world we live in, it's worth a try.

5

. . . . .

Handcrafted Babies

Recently, I had the opportunity to sit in a two-tone Phantom Zenith Rolls-Royce convertible. Historically, I haven't been much of a car person, but to sit behind the wheel and revel in the exquisite craftsmanship of this car was, I must confess, a complete thrill! Every detail of the car exudes intelligence, wisdom, and a style that invites envy.

The Phantom represents the pinnacle of driving elegance. Each car is handmade, with only fifty individual models of the one I sat in built each year. The manufacturer's suggested retail price starts at $492,000, but the model I got to sit in goes for upward of $650,000—*which is why I was only allowed to sit in it and not drive it!*

How We Should Construct Our Children

If luxury automobiles are constructed slowly, intentionally, and by hand, I contend we should also skillfully raise our children with the same devotion. And we should start from the very moment they are born. The good news for moms and dads is your sons and daughters are primed and ready for the challenge. Studies show that the one hundred billion neurons that your babies are born with are already astir: ripe for shaping, poised to be molded, and imprinting virtually all that they encounter.

This is where parenting comes into the equation. The top priority for new moms and dads is to *be there* and shepherd their children as they grow. Raising emotionally and intellectually healthy children doesn't happen by chance in a vacuum. It requires thoughtful parental oversight. Babies who thrive need parents who are willing to make the sacrifice to "handcraft" and attach to them *right from the start*.

The Birth of Attachment Theory

Researchers John Bowlby and Mary Ainsworth, working in the mid-twentieth century, studied the importance of early relationships between parents or other caretakers and young children. After extensive study, they uncovered findings that still rock and challenge our world. Their work would later become known as *attachment theory*.

After countless hours of observing babies with their mothers and fathers, they found that focused attention from parents—or other committed caregivers—in the first weeks and months of a newborn's life had a lasting impact on how the children they studied later turned out. What Bowlby and Ainsworth found was concentrated and loving adult input into the lives of their young children wasn't wasted romanticism or wanton doting. In fact, "handcrafted" children turned out better.

Their research—and the studies of the many others who followed them—proved that children who, from early on, have loving, caring, and consistently involved parents *thrive* in mind and body. Their brains are physically *larger* in size (they score higher on IQ exams too), they exhibit more stability emotionally, and even their physical health is more robust.

Bowlby wrote in 1953 that "the quality of the parental care which a child receives in his earliest years is of *vital importance for his future mental health* [italics added]." From his work researching maternal-child relationships over fifty years, Bowlby concluded that intense love in the early days of children's lives makes a critical difference in how they ultimately feel about themselves and how they relate to the world around them. As he put it, "The way parents treat a child . . . is of key importance in determining [their] development."

Mary Ainsworth, Bowlby's attachment theory codeveloper, wrote in the early 1940s: "Familial security in the early stages . . . forms a basis from which the individual can work out gradually, forming new skills and interests in other fields." In other words, children, from the very beginning, need a stable and supportive foundation from which to explore the world around them.

That secure base from which children venture off into the world *is their parents*. Knowing there are adults who love them, children have the freedom to explore and become creative. They venture out because they know that there is a solid refuge to return to and caring guardians who are watching and championing their every foray.

One Special Bond

Another one of Bowlby's signature theories was *monotropy*. Bowlby posited that for an infant to properly develop, he needs the loving care of *one* individual who is kind and reliable; a *life partner* who is there for him. Historically, this person has been the child's mother, but circumstances don't always afford this convenient arrangement. In such cases, other individuals who are affectionate, focused, stable, and committed to the child, such as family members—fathers, grandmothers, aunts—or long-term, loving, and attentive nannies, can act as surrogates. These substitute caretakers are as effective as a mother in developing healthy attachment and socialization in a child.

Bowlby referred to these individuals as *attachment figures* who functioned as surrogate mothers, but he went on to warn that these individuals *must* maintain their relationship with the child for years to ensure emotional stability and tranquility. Early loss of a surrogate can result in the child experiencing the same traumatic loss that a child experiences by the early or untimely loss of a parent.

Attachment Timetable

Bowlby also demonstrated that there was a time window during which attachment was critical. He pegged the first eighteen to twenty-four months of life as the critical period for mothers (or attachment figures) to be intimately involved with the child. From his observations of mothers with their children, he concluded that physical and mental development could only proceed smoothly if babies enjoy a loving and enduring figure during these first early months.

For the first two years of their lives, babies need people around who touch them, talk and sing to them, swing them high in the air, laugh with them, massage them, stroke their cheeks, and glory in their first smiles. Their early coos need to be answered by someone who loves them dearly. Their guttural baby growls require a reciprocating response. Their newborn neurons need to be wooed. Babies need to know that they are loved. They glory in warm snuggles, soothing voices, and fervent prayers. This is what attachment theory is all about.

More Than Milk

Bowlby's theories were buttressed by the work of Harry Harlow, a psychologist best known for his studies in maternal deprivation and dependency. In now famous experiments, Harlow took newborn infant rhesus monkeys from their natural mothers at birth and put them into cages with nonliving, wire mother surrogates. One wire mommy held an inverted milk bottle from which the infant monkey could feed. The other wire mother surrogate was wrapped in a soft terry cloth towel but provided no milk to the baby monkey.

What Harlow found was this: baby monkeys would suckle and feed from the wire surrogate with the milk bottle, but when they were done, they would scurry back to the terry cloth surrogate to snuggle.

The interaction between these young monkeys and the milk-dispensing surrogate mother and the terry cloth–covered surrogate mother, who did not deliver any milk, demonstrated that baby monkeys needed and wanted more from a mother than just milk: they needed a mother who was soft, a mother who they could cozy up to.

Human babies are not monkey babies. They are more capable of adapting, but Harlow's experiments hinted at a pattern that is undeniable: primates crave nurturing as much as they need nutrition.

The relevance of Harlow's work to humans was borne out by a 2014 study of premature babies who were required to spend weeks or even months in newborn intensive care units. Babies who were touched during their prolonged hospitalization developed quicker with fewer complications than those who were not. Specifically, babies who had skin-to-skin contact with their mothers showed better cognitive skills when they were tested even ten years later.

Round-the-Clock Parenting

A distinction between attachment theory, as developed by Bowlby and others, and *attachment parenting* is in order. Attachment parenting takes attachment theory to a different level and maintains that secure connections between mother and baby require continuous, 24-7 physical contact.

I don't recommend this kind of intense parenting model because I don't think it's reasonable, nor do I think it is necessary. Attachment parenting takes attachment theory concepts, which are grounded on solid research, to an unacceptable extreme.

The Nonattached

Bowlby categorized children who never experience loving one-on-one acceptance and care on a consistent basis from an adult figure as *nonattached*. Unlike children who grow up in loving and warm families, these children are at high risk for irreversible emotional, social, and intellectual problems.

Studies published in the mid-twentieth century looked at children who were separated from their parents at an early age during the Nazis' bombing blitz of London during World War II, as well as other children who were likewise separated from their parents early in their lives. The studies showed that both groups of young boys and girls didn't do well. They suffered immense emotional lability both as children and later as adults.

The researchers from this study concluded that these individuals, who had endured such disruptive experiences as young children and who never had the opportunity to adequately attach to a parent figure, started out life unformed and broken. As they aged, they tended toward higher levels of delinquency, aggression, and social awkwardness, and as adults, they were unable to form meaningful relationships with others.

Forty-Four Thieves

In 1944, John Bowlby published yet another seminal article that he entitled "Forty-Four Juvenile Thieves." In it, he reported his findings on studying the early years of a group of young children and teenagers who habitually robbed those around them. What he found was that many of these young thieves had experienced highly dysfunctional and disrupted childhoods. Several were raised in *foundling homes* (orphanages for newborns), and others bounced from one foster home to another during their first few years of life.

Bowlby concluded that the forty-four "thieves" he studied were *nonattached people* who never knew consistent and genuine love during the first months to years of their lives. They were "hollow" people who bumped along in life at the fringes, indifferent to true love and incapable of deep human relationships.

The High Price of Separation

Motivated by Bowlby's groundbreaking work, in 1949, the newly formed World Health Organization (WHO) asked Bowlby to write a report on mental health conditions of homeless children. After several months of international study, Bowlby produced a report called *Maternal Care and Mental Health*, in which he stated, "What goes on in the internal world is more or less an accurate reflection of what an individual has experienced in the external world."

He went on to say that "separation experiences"—deprivation of mothers during the first twelve to eighteen months of life—are "pathogenic." In other words, he found that children who didn't have a loving attachment figure during the first critical months of their young lives tended toward psychological maladies. These children were at higher risk for both mental and physical illnesses, including personality disorders, anxiety disorders, and a "psychopathic personality," which meant they tended toward mental illness. To Bowlby, it was clear: loving caretakers who meet the emotional needs of an infant, *beyond* just the provision of food, make the crucial difference in the lives of children, both short term and long term.

As Bowlby put it, what was essential for robust mental health was that "the infant and young child . . . experience a warm, intimate and continuous relationship with his mother (or mother-substitute), in which *both* [my emphasis] find satisfaction and enjoyment. A child needs to feel he is an object of pleasure and pride to his mother; a mother needs to feel an expansion of her own personality in the personality of her child: each need to feel closely identified with the other."

Institutionalized Children

Bowlby and Ainsworth built their attachment theory not only from their own intimate experiences with families in England, America, and Uganda but also on the work of others from earlier in the twentieth century who had evaluated the prevailing care that institutionalized infants received in hospitals, foundling homes, and orphanages.

In the late nineteenth and early twentieth century, the thinking about children was very different from the way it is today. It was a colder and sterner world for children in those times. The adage "children are to be seen, but not heard" was the norm.

Despite anecdotal evidence that maternal separation was

harmful, hospitals in the early twentieth century ignored this evidence and separated parents from children during prolonged illnesses. The thinking at the time was hospitals were to be sanitary and sterile environments, off-limits to anyone who could be a potential source of germs. Children who were admitted to a hospital during these days were forbidden visits from parents or other family members for fear that visitors would bring infectious agents into patients' rooms.

While in the hospital, these children were also restricted in their contact with the staff for fear that such contact would, likewise, harm their health. As a result, some young children were held in hospitals and tragically deprived of parental love and staff contact for months at a time.

This same wrongheaded and nonsensical reasoning was applied to orphaned children as well. Institutions at that time provided food, clothing, and a clean environment for their orphans, but intimate, warm relationships between staff and children were discouraged. It was assumed that these young babies would soon be adopted, so any intimacy would be damaging since it would be only short term. Unfortunately, this was not always the case. Many children spent *years* in "sanitary" facilities that were indifferent and emotionally cold and where they received, *by intention*, little to no human contact.

The outcome of this "care" was appalling. These warehoused children, who were raised with restricted and inconsistent human contact, were markedly delayed. When compared to children who had been adopted out early or others who had been placed in foster homes, they were intellectually slow and had strikingly lower IQs.

They also died early. In a study of children under one year of age admitted to ten institutions in the United Kingdom during 1915, 32–75 percent (depending on the institution) died by the end of their second year of care.

The explanations that doctors gave for this phenomenon were vague at best. They were at a loss to explain these astronomical mortality rates and put them down to hospitalism, institutionalism, or failure to thrive. None of these adequately explained what was going on. Looking back, it's quite clear; these children died from broken hearts. They died because they were deprived of human love and human contact. They died because no one was addressing their emotional needs. Babies need more than three meals a day and a crib; they need consistent and loving care from another human being.

Another researcher, René Spitz, also studied children suffering from hospitalism and found, like Bowlby and Ainsworth, that young children who were deprived of mothering during the first two years of life were not only damaged as children, they were also unable to form healthy connections with people as they aged. Their behavioral abnormalities persisted even when they were later placed in loving and caring adoptive and foster homes. Unfortunately, the damage had already been done. These children were permanently affected, and the amount of impairment was directly related to the level of their deprivation during their early years.

Spitz found that the injury to these children was evident in *all* areas of development. Babies who were institutionalized in impersonal and sterile environments during the first two years of life deteriorated to the point of being stuporous and nonresponsive to human faces. Spitz wrote, "If between the sixth and eighteenth months of life an infant is deprived of its mother without adequate substitute, [the child's] development becomes retarded in the course of the first two months of separation. It becomes increasingly unapproachable, weepy and screaming."

He later documented this rapid developmental deterioration in a silent movie that he released in 1952. It showed children suffering from what he called *psychogenic diseases in infancy* and became the source of great consternation in the psychological community. One viewer later wrote that Spitz's movie was "one of the little-known horror films of our time." I've watched this archived film. It is utterly heartbreaking to see a previously normal child descend into bleak silence due to emotional deprivation.

The observations of hospitalism are really nothing new. A Spanish bishop who worked with orphans two centuries earlier wrote in his personal journal that the abandoned children he attempted to care for became profoundly "sad and many of them die from sadness."

More recently, researcher Harry Chugani, M.D., studied a group of post–Cold War Romanian children who had been adopted by U.S. families from orphanages that also functioned on the century-old paradigm of limited contact between child and caregiver. Using functional MRI (fMRI), Chugani demonstrated that the brains of the emotionally and physically deprived Romanian children were smaller and less complex neurologically than normal controls, thus proving visually that young babies who don't have loving care in the first years of life suffer irreparable neurological harm.

Attachment Theory Is Pro-Parent

The ideas of Bowlby and Ainsworth were controversial when they were first published nearly sixty-five years ago, and they continue to ruffle feathers today. To the Freudian-based psychoanalysts of that time, who based much of their understanding of children on retrospective extrapolations and inferences from their adult patients, *behavioral psychology*, which is based on actual observations of children and the foundation of attachment theory, was foreign territory. Attachment theory didn't fit their mold, and thus, they never fully embraced nor did they care to understand what Bowlby and Ainsworth had uncovered.

The psychoanalysts weren't alone in their criticism of Bowlby and Ainsworth. Feminists, later in the century, likewise took aim at attachment theory. To the feminists, attachment theory was hostile scientific evidence that tied women more fervently to the hearth, at least during their child-rearing years.

Even today, with an increasing number of women in the workforce and many new mothers returning to work within months (or even weeks) after giving birth, the findings of Bowlby and Ainsworth still stoke strong emotions. It's not difficult to understand why they represented a frontal attack on nonmaternal childcare.

Quotes like this one from Bowlby only add fuel to the fire:

This whole business of mothers going to work, it's so bitterly controversial, but I do not think it's a good idea. I mean women go out to work and make some daffily [*sic*] little bit of gadgetry which has no particular social value, and children are looked after in indifferent day nurseries.

It's very difficult to get people to look after other people's children. Looking after your own children is hard work. But you get some rewards in that. Looking after other people's children is very hard work, and you don't get many rewards for it. I think that the role of parents has been grossly undervalued, crassly undervalued. All the emphasis has been put on so-called economic prosperity.

As one may expect, Bowlby's inflammatory comments led to furious debate, but, despite his insensitive delivery, attachment theory proponents have stood firm on the *research* of Bowlby and Ainsworth and even today contend that it doesn't "take a village" to raise a child; it only takes one committed individual.

Opponents, looking to undermine attachment theory, angrily and oddly began to even devalue the awareness and innate intellect of newborns, along with the importance of one-on-one adult-infant relationships during the first months to years of life. One professor was quoted in a 1987 *Time* magazine article as saying that newborn babies have "brains [that] are Jell-O and . . . memories akin to those of decorticate rodents." This unseemly comment, and others like it, trivialized the neurological sophistication of young infants. If newborn babies are passive lumps who have no cognitive awareness, why should parents bother with them at all?

But this was never true. Ask any mother if her child is a "Jellohead" and you will get a strong response. And with the advent of fMRIs, scientists can now *see* and document *in living color* the growth and development of a child's brain from the very early days of life.

Opponents of attachment theory also set out to tarnish the halo that surrounds babies and their parents—a loving and committed relationship that researchers had proved years earlier as being of utmost importance to the newborn. They also sought to belittle bonding and the value of the roles mothers and fathers play in the first few days and weeks with their newborn babies. One outspoken critic of attachment theory believed that a child's social and intellectual development was "rendered nearly invulnerable by biological design." In other words, according to this critic, no matter what happens in a newborn's life, everything is in the DNA. Genetics trump environment.

But current evidence shows that critic got it wrong. When it comes to genetics versus environment, the debate is over: they are both important.

In the presence of a supportive environment, an attached primary caregiver, and a healthy diet, the brain typically thrives.

—AMERICAN ACADEMY OF PEDIATRICS STATEMENT ON THE
FIRST ONE THOUSAND DAYS OF NUTRITION, 2018

Genes Versus the Environment

Genes clearly play an important role in the overall health and abilities of a child. As one example, children who are born with genetic defects such as Down syndrome have lower IQs than babies without Down syndrome.

But equally important is the part environment plays in the well-being of children. For example, babies who are malnourished or babies whose *mothers* were malnourished during their pregnancies don't thrive, and studies show that their overall mental abilities are compromised. Likewise, babies who are born into emotional deprivation also suffer irreparable harm.

On the other hand, children who are raised in enriched, emotionally healthy homes with caring and concerned caretakers win. It is estimated that the IQs of children who enjoy such advantaged circumstances are enhanced by twenty to thirty points.

SURPRISE: You can boost your babies' IQs by loving them more.

A Word About Childcare

Whether people like them or not, childcare centers are here to stay. Mothers are returning to the workforce in full-time employment positions earlier and earlier after giving birth. Based on Department of Labor figures from 2012, about 23 percent of women—nearly one in four—were back at work within two weeks of delivering their babies. These women often (though not always) need childcare to continue their work outside of their homes.

This creates an enormous demand for childcare services, and

over the past several years, childcare has evolved into a sizable service industry.

The Effect of the Wrong Kind of Childcare

But what are the effects of nonmaternal care of children in the early months and years of life? Researcher Dr. Jay Belsky has done extensive research concerning this issue. His studies show that children who spend their early years in nonmaternal childcare that is extensive (twenty hours or more per week), who are enrolled in childcare young (less than one year of life), and whose childcare is of poor quality (understaffed and unstimulating centers that are unresponsive to verbal or nonverbal cues from the child and that do not render warm and supportive care to the child) tend to be more aggressive and more noncompliant than children who spent their early years with their mothers.

That said, all day cares are not created equal. Robert Karen, author of *Becoming Attached* and a scholar on attachment theory, told me in a personal communication that high-quality, responsive day care can be enriching for children, particularly in the development of social skills. He warns, however, against putting children into day care too early. He recommends that parents wait at least six months before they place their children into a day-care facility.

Dr. Bob's Recommendations for the First Year

So how do working moms and dads navigate childcare in the first year? This is a question that creates serious anxiety for the parents I care for in my practice. Here are my recommendations.

If it is at all possible, I recommend that mothers spend the entire first year home with their newborns. The research bears out that this is a giant bonus for your baby and also brings joy and a sense of tranquility to mothers and fathers alike.

I know for many couples, this is an unreasonable stretch. Many families face financial challenges that make this option simply impossible. Women with professional careers, and without legislated maternal leave protection, like those found in many European countries, have a difficult time extracting themselves from their responsibilities for this length of time. But with these and other considerations in mind, I still think considering taking an entire year with your baby, away from the fray of the workplace, is best. It will take some hard-nosed negotiations with the company you work for and some serious financial planning and budgeting, but it's worth a try.

If a year is not possible, take full advantage of your maternity leave, then tack on every extra vacation and sick day you have accrued to extend your time with your new son or daughter.

> **SURPRISE:** Many European countries have very generous parental leave laws. New parents in Sweden, for instance, are entitled to 480 days of leave at 80 percent of their normal pay.

When you finally do go back to work, try to negotiate an abbreviated schedule and ask if you can do some of your work from home. In our connected, internet-driven world, this is becoming more and more of a viable option for many of the mothers in my practice.

And finally, all this advice *also* applies to fathers. If you have a liberal paternity policy at your place of employment, take full advantage of it. Chisel out as much time as you possibly can to be with your baby. Between moms and dads, families are often able to piece together a significant stretch of time when your baby is cared for by one of you. This is good news for your baby, since you are the ones your baby has bonded to best.

Finding Childcare for the First Year

Finally, if you cannot spend a full year away from your work, see what you can do to find a family member, like a grandmother or aunt, to come to your home and care for your newborn. Family members are generally invested in your child as much as you are. A loving grandmother may be the best possible caretaker your child would ever have. I know this personally because I see the loving care my wife provides for our grandchildren.

If finding a close relative is also not feasible, then for the first year, I recommend hiring a responsible nanny to come to your home. This is generally more expensive than traditional day care, but since year one is such an important period for your child both developmentally and emotionally, it's worth the cost.

One final thought: when you hire a nanny, you must hire a "you equivalent." Remember what you are doing. You're finding someone to replace *you* to care for your child. So the nanny you hire can't just be good, he or she must be excellent. This will be a challenge because the nanny your child needs is one who will go the extra mile, someone who will fall as desperately in love with your baby as you have, and someone who will love and bond with your baby as deeply and profoundly as you have.

Young Babies Get Sick

One final reason I like to see babies home for the first year is being home minimizes a child's exposure to illnesses. Day cares, no matter how fastidious or assiduous they are, find it next to impossible to prevent sick kids from coming to their facilities. Children are simply too dynamic medically for parents or day-care workers to know when they are getting sick. A child can wake up in the morning and appear to be fine, but within hours he can spike a fever. Exposure to viral infections is part of the deal when parents put their children into a day-care center, no matter the size of the facility. Even smaller, house-based centers deal with these same challenges.

Children kept at home, on the other hand, away from the general community, tend to be healthier for the first year than those who are enrolled in day care. For working mothers and fathers, healthier babies translates into fewer days away from the office to care for your sick child.

Babies Need Love!

Bowlby and Ainsworth's work from the 1950s and the many studies from then until today all confirm something that we all intrinsically already know—namely, *young babies need an abundance of love*. They need devoted, handcrafted attention from the moment they are born, and they need it consistently, especially during the early years of their lives. When children are born, parents are called upon to provide them with the love that they need. Parenting is a high calling, but it has never been easy. Planning ahead, making hard decisions, and factoring in adequate time to intensively parent your baby will contribute, in the long term, to a healthier and more emotionally stable child.

6

. . . . .

Four Cornerstones of the First Year

Secret #4: Solid and Healthy Families Don't Happen by Chance—They Are Created with Deliberation

On July 4, 1848, fifteen thousand people gathered in Washington, D.C., to witness the laying of the cornerstone of a monument that would ultimately be the world's tallest obelisk, a towering spire that would honor and memorialize the commander in chief of the Continental Army and America's first president, George Washington. The stone weighed 24,500 pounds, and the moment was one of great ceremony. One speaker, Joseph R. Chandler, said of Washington, "No more Washingtons shall come in our time . . . but his virtues are stamped on the heart of mankind."

Cornerstones are ceremoniously placed into the foundations of buildings inscribed with the date construction began, the names of prominent individuals involved in the building, or the name of the institution that will occupy the building, and they usually include the architects who created the structure.

More important, however, is their position in the building and the value this plays in construction. Cornerstones are perfectly placed and trued in all measurements because, as construction proceeds, they serve as *reference points* and determine the position of the rest of structure.

Cornerstones represent the strength and the architectural fidelity of a building, and thus, cornerstone placement, beyond the ceremony, pomp, and circumstance that accompany the moment, is a careful, deliberate, and *serious* act. Wise parents—those who want to raise healthy and emotionally stable children—must likewise consciously establish and build upon the cornerstones that will be their reference points for their family.

What Are the Touchstones That Will Govern Your Family?

So what will be the cornerstones, those essential elements, that will guide your family? These questions are important and, from my observation of young couples, rarely asked. But they should be, and I believe they fall into the following four categories:

1. What do we believe?
2. What kind of parents are we going to be?
3. What community do we belong to?
4. How will we care for our child's health?

1. The Cornerstone of Faith

From one generation to the next may we declare your greatness, and for all eternity may we affirm your holiness. And, may our praise, oh God, never be absent from our

> *mouths, now and forever. For you are a great and holy God.*
> *Blessed are you, the Awesome One, the Holy God.*
>
> —BAR MITZVAH BOOKLET

You're Gonna Serve Somebody

The 2016 Nobel Prize winner for literature, singer Bob Dylan, once wrote a song entitled "Gotta Serve Somebody." The thesis of his song is that human beings need to believe in somebody or something to anchor their lives.

The lyrics of his song were poignant, and his conclusion was blunt: "It may be the devil or it may be the Lord, but you're gonna have to *serve* somebody!" For Dylan, we all have a choice to make; either we'll embrace the light or we'll end up chasing the dark.

Dylan was right. There's an inexplicable *something* down deep in our DNA that affirms Dylan's proposition. Look around the world. Anywhere and everywhere you find humans, you will also find belief systems that govern their lives. Embedded in the human soul is a void that causes us to look up and seek something bigger and grander than ourselves. Babies have this proclivity too.

Our Spiritual Babies

In her book *The Spiritual Child*, Lisa Miller, Ph.D., writes: "Spirituality is . . . part of our natural endowment, just like our abilities to see, smell and think." She goes on to say that people are "inherently, genetically spiritual." This "genetic expression of spirituality surges in adolescence," and "our natural spirituality is allied closely with human bonding."

For many, contemplating these kinds of existential questions brings discomfort. Spiritual reflection and introspection is not a part of our modern-day modus operandi. And yet when a child is born, even secular, nonbelieving individuals look at the event as miraculous, supernatural, and awe-inspiring. I have personally witnessed many deliveries, and there's a profound, unspoken sense of the sacred when a newborn child draws its first breath.

My Journey in the Faith

I was raised in a strong Christian family. My father, a hardworking and, in his day, hard-living, former U.S. Navy, former Merchant Marine, tough guy converted to the Christian faith in his mid-thirties. My mother also converted to the faith, and subsequently, their lives radically changed, as did their parenting goals. We became a churchgoing family, and through their example, my parents successfully passed their faith on to all five of their children. Even today, all my siblings are practicing, Bible-believing followers of Jesus.

For me, my faith rescued me from indecision and a lot of other potential pitfalls. I knew what I believed from an early age, and this provided the touchstone from which I evaluated the ideas and events around me. I had a sense of destiny (God loved me and cared about me) that brought clarity to my life and shielded me from drugs, sex, and delinquency. I understood, even as a young child, that some behaviors were wrong and other things were right in the eyes of God. I have never regretted my decision to continue in the faith and will forever thank my parents for the spiritual moorings that they passed on to me.

With these spiritual roots in my life, my wife and I have likewise raised our children in a Christian community in Southern California, which has provided for them a warm, enriching, and supportive environment to grow. From the very beginning, we hoped to hand off to them the spiritual virtues of kindness, love, gratitude, and forgiveness. We desired (and still do) that each of our children have a deep and abiding love for the Lord and a solid understanding of the spiritual dimension of life.

Prayers for Our Babies

Even when our children were babies, my wife and I prayed for and with them. We taught them that there was a loving God who watched over the affairs of men and had a perfect plan for their lives.

Praying with an infant child may not seem like a particularly productive exercise to some. Your children certainly do not understand the content of your words, but they do capture a sense of hope, reverence, and warmth when you invoke the name of God. Praying for our children also reminds us (and I am talking about *we* who are praying) of the glory and the miracle of the little lives we hold in our hands. Our prayers also cause us to remember our sense of duty, before God, to our children.

Leslie and I are not alone in our desires. I know many others who desire that their children follow their lead in faith. The spiritual life of your child is important, even from the very beginning. A clear and unclouded faith in God yields great blessings throughout life, so don't wait to expose this dimension to your child. Pray with them and encourage them frequently—and start when they are young. Spiritual foundations in your family are important and should be cultivated.

2. The Cornerstone of Parenting

Are we ever truly *ready* to be parents? The nine months of gestation are a primer, a preparation for about-to-be-parents, but I think the answer to the question is clearly *no!* Nobody is *really* ready, even when labor begins.

But at the very instant your little angel is born, something astounding occurs and—guess what?—*you're now ready!*

Most moms and dads immediately rise to the challenge. Just like baby, they have their own birth experience. They're birthed into parenthood.

Go Look in the Mirror

Since parenting is a big undertaking, shortly after a child is born, I frequently tell parents to start talking to themselves. "Go find a mirror," I advise them, "and tell yourself—out loud—that you are a parent." This may seem like an odd recommendation, but I encourage this exercise because parenthood is a role that can so overwhelm young new moms and dads that it takes verbal and mental practice to feel comfortable wearing the title. Telling your friend that the child you're walking around with is your daughter or son will initially sound strange. The words almost stick in your mouth. To gain some fluency, you've got to practice. So go find yourself a mirror and start a conversation, because the role of a parent is bigger and more important than almost anything else you will ever do.

There is another reason why I want new parents to talk in the mirror to themselves. I don't want parents to think, even for a moment, that they are their children's friends or confidants.

They are neither, even from the beginning.

Babies need parents.

Consider this for a moment. Think about your own parents. Ponder the relationship you had or currently have with them. Now consider the relationship you had or currently have with your best friend or your partner or your siblings. Are they not all totally different relationships? Of course, parents can be friendly with their children, but the primary work of parents is to guide and shape, encourage and nurture, as well as discipline their children and hold them to high standards. Being friends or confidants can get in the way of these primary goals. So get it right from the start. You are your child's parent.

> ## Be the Kind of Parent Who Talks to Your Children
>
> Studies show that moms and dads who talk to their children and interact with them in a positive way—as parents—will have children who will, more likely, during their teenage years talk to them about the worries and challenges they face.

How Do We Do It Right?

Writer and talk radio host Laura Schlessinger put it this way: you have two opportunities in life to get it right when it comes to parent-child relationships. The first opportunity (between you and your parents) you have little to no control over. The second opportunity (between you and your children) you have *total* control over.

If your first parent-child relationship was stellar, you were fortunate. You've received an invaluable gift, and it will serve you well as you venture forth into parenthood. If your first parent-child interaction was not optimal, however, this can be hobbling because, for better or worse, how we respond to our children often reflects how our own parents raised us. This is what I call our *fallback position*.

John Bowlby said it well when he wrote, "The roots of parenthood lie in the child's relations to his own parents in his earliest years. The love which a mother has for her children is a reflection of the love which she received when she was a little girl. The love which a father has for his children is a reflection of the love which he received when he was a little boy. It is in childhood that we learn to love."

But nothing is indelibly etched into our nature. People do have the ability to change and overcome their go-to, fallback tendencies. In my work with families, I have seen many parents in action. Not one of them is perfect, because there are no perfect people, but there are general concepts that yield good fruit. The parents in my practice who have *won* the parenting prize are those who are loving, kind, gracious, sensitive, and firm.

Finding the Right Balance

Diana Baumrind, Ph.D., a psychologist who studies parenting styles, has found that the optimal parent is one who is simultaneously loving and strict. Yes, you can be loving and strict at the same time. Some of my most memorable and best teachers were kind and gracious people, but they also enforced the rules. They drew a line, and when push came to shove, they were unyielding.

Expanding on Baumrind's work, researchers E. E. Maccoby and J. A. Martin described four parenting styles that were based on two criteria: *responsiveness* (acceptance) and *demandingness* (control). Responsiveness parents were defined as those parents who intentionally promoted "individuality, self-regulation and self-assertion." Responsiveness parents are also accepting parents who are "supportive of a child's needs and demands."

Demandingness parents, on the other hand, were defined as those parents who supervised, disciplined, and confronted their children when they disobeyed. Demandingness parents are controlling parents who oversee the affairs of their children with vigilance and demand obedience to the rules.

Four Parenting Styles

From these two parameters, they identified four parenting styles:

1. *Authoritarian* style parents rank high in demandingness but fall shy when it comes to responsiveness to their children. These parents are sometimes referred to as totalitarian.

2. *Authoritative* parents also rank high in demandingness and rank high in responsiveness as well.

3. *Permissive* or *indulgent* parents rank low in demandingness and high in responsiveness.

4. Finally, *negligent* parents rank low in both categories. Negligent parents don't make any demands on their children and don't really engage their children either. In essence, they neglect their children because they don't seem to care one way or another what their children are doing.

It should come as no surprise that the sweet spot for parenting types is the *authoritative* style. Their studies showed that parents who were demanding but loving and responsive to their children produced offspring who performed better in society. Children raised in authoritative homes have a better understanding of how things work. They follow the rules and succeed at higher levels than children raised in authoritarian, indulgent, or negligent homes. This is the balance parents should strive for.

Hands-On Versus Hands-Off Parenting

Another question you must ask yourself is whether you are going to be a *hands-on* or *hands-off* parent. My advice is this: be both. Usually, what your children need to do is figure things out for themselves—and this even applies to young babies.

When your daughter is attempting to roll over, for example, let her work through the struggle of doing it. There's a technique in rolling over, and it is important that your girl, through trial and error, find the right way to do it. It's tempting to reach out and help her with a gentle nudge, but resist those good intentions! Let her struggle through it. Jumping in and fixing things will only inhibit your daughter's growth toward independence and self-confidence.

The frustration of not being able to do something isn't always bad. It drives us forward. When babies and young children finally achieve their goal, they sense that they have achieved something significant, so don't mess with the process.

On the other hand, when your children are learning something new, they do need teaching. Teaching is a hands-on process. We learn by watching something being done and hearing how to do it and then by attempting it ourselves. That is what education is all about.

When I was a young boy, my father taught me how to tie a necktie. I remember looking in the mirror and trying to make my mirror-inverted fingers follow his instruction. It was a painful and thoroughly frustrating process. He was patient, however, and at times put his hands over mine to help me loop the tie correctly. In time, I learned how to do it, but it took his instruction—including his hands over mine—for me to ultimately figure it out. This is hands-on learning at its best.

During my training in pediatrics—another apprenticeship-like, hands-on experience—we learned and followed the adage "Watch one, do one, teach one." This meant that after we had watched a particular procedure being done, it was then time for us to do one, and finally, in order to etch this new skill into our brains, we had to likewise teach it to someone else.

With your babies, learn to be parents who both actively watch their children struggle through an experience and who actively teach their children with hands-on instruction. When to employ passive observation verses active teaching is a matter of judgment. This is the reason parenting is called an art. There are no hard-and-fast rules, but you get better as the days go by.

Helicopterish Behaviors

Overattentive helicoptering as a parental style is a manifestation of inner anxiety and a lack of faith. Children are very sensitive to this "nervous Nellie" kind of parenting and often react like everyone else reacts: with avoidance and disdain. As writer and professor Jordan B. Peterson puts it, "Too much protection devastates the soul."

So if you tend to fuss over details and are given to hovering over your children, stop now! Give them some breathing room. Micromanaging your children is never a good tactic, and it rarely works.

For those compulsive souls who can't rein in their jittery tendencies, I recommend that they hurry out and have four or five more children as soon as possible. Having a brood of children at your feet cures all helicoptering because nobody has that kind of energy or time to hover over them all!

Free-Spirited or Plan-Ahead Approach

Are you a free-spirited or a plan-ahead kind of person? When it comes to parenting, both free-spirited and plan-ahead parenting styles have benefits.

Those who plan carefully have fewer surprises, but there is something delightful in those spontaneous moments where, without long deliberation, parents do something wild. Grabbing your kids and taking them to the beach on the spur of the moment—even on a day they are supposed to be in school—yields some of the most wonderful moments and memories your children will ever have. This applies to your less-than-one-year-old-baby too!

When it comes to parenting, you've also got to plan ahead, but every so often, let yourself do something that no one will expect you to do—and do it with your children.

Tiger Moms

And finally, for those tiger moms and dads who push their children ever onward to participate in mammoth athletic or musical endeavors—restrain yourselves. Change your aggressive ways before it is too late. Put down those flash cards for your four-month-old baby, and allow your child the time to relax and soak in her environment.

Parents were never meant to be talent agents. They're called to nurture and encourage.

Too Much of a Good Thing

I had a patient once whose father was determined that his son play professional basketball. Day in and day out, with nary a break, this unfortunate lad was forced to practice the fundamentals of the game with his pushy father and an assortment of private coaches. Home was a never-ending basketball camp that never allowed this young boy the opportunity to discover who he was and what *he* wanted to do.

I repeatedly warned the father that it was too much, but he ignored my advice.

During elementary school, this young man was indeed a sensational standout on the basketball court, but when he progressed into junior high school, he wearied of the program and simply quit, to the great disappointment of this father. He wasn't a bad kid, but he wasn't a machine, and when he was old enough to push back, he was done with the gig. And all the time and money the father had put into his son's basketball career were lost.

3. The Cornerstone of Community

The word *community* is derived from the Latin word *communis*, which means "things held in common." A community is a group, small or large, that shares values, norms, and a locality. It may be a village or a neighborhood, a church, a work environment, or even a club.

Your home is going to be the first community your child will know. The home you create should abound in warmth, hope, and love. Edmund Burke once wrote, "We begin our public affections in our families." Our homes should be nurturing, kind, and fun environments where responsibilities are shared and where the friendship and love between a child's parents is palpable. This "outer womb" that we share with our babies is the foundation from which our children build their lives and understand greater community.

The layers of the community onion, beyond your nuclear family, are likewise important. Children who grow up in a rich tapestry of relationships—grandparents, uncles, aunts, cousins, and non-related friends and acquaintances—have a deeper sense of belonging than those who live their lives separated from others. There's also a larger community, beyond our individual homes and families that we want to expose our children to as well.

What does this mean? Simply this: if you were hanging out with a group of people before you have a baby, double down and keep hanging out with them after you have your baby. If you were regulars at the corner deli every Friday night before you were parents, when your baby gets old enough to get out of the house (about one month of age), get yourself back down to the deli on Friday night.

Disappearing People

I have seen couples who drop off the face of the earth after they have babies. Before children, they were a part of a vibrant and active community of friends, but after their babies arrived, they disappeared into the intergalactic ether—no traces left except soiled diapers. This parched, shut-in social status is usually prompted by fear of infection or a self-imposed need to slavishly follow their children's schedules.

To me, this is sad. And not at all necessary.

Here is how I see it: When you become a parent, you will need to make a lot of changes to accommodate the new little person in your life, but the responsibility to adapt should not rest on your shoulders alone.

Your baby needs to make accommodations too.

You read that right. Your baby needs to get with the program! And if you give him the opportunity, he will. Never underestimate the malleability of children, and don't be intimidated by unwritten rules telling parents that they need to adhere to rigid schedules and feeding times. Life is messier than that, and there should be a little reciprocity in this new relationship. If you lean in toward your babies, expect and require that they lean in toward you too.

I understand this may read harshly, but it is unquestionably true. Parents who eternally defer to their children, even young babies, are spoiling them and setting themselves up for problems in the future.

So keep your friends close, embrace your community, keep playing an active role in what you were doing before your baby came into your life, and bring your baby with you. He will benefit from the interaction—and you will too, as you will find your community wants to participate with you in raising your child.

Children in the Community

I have been to Africa more than twenty times, leading medical missions to underdeveloped countries, including Sierra Leone, Liberia, and Tanzania. While there caring for the children of these countries, I have received an up-close-and-personal tutorial on the interaction between African mothers, their babies, and the broader community.

Here is what I have learned: African babies are with their mothers all the time! As their mothers manage the business of day-to-day life, the babies are strapped to their mothers' backs and go with them everywhere—into the marketplace, into the fields, and onto ridiculously crowded buses.

Not sequestered from the vibrancy of the community at home or in day-care crannies, babies are a part of the living organism we call *community* from the very start. It's a seamless life for these children, and they contribute to the colorful, generationally blurred, vibrant quilt that is the African community. Far from being excluded, children are right in the middle of the ebb and flow of the adult workaday world, taking it in, learning from it all, and enriching it.

Freshness and Delight

Children bring a freshness and delight to the marketplace. Screaming babies are commonly encountered in the day-to-day African culture. I find this is all wonderful and quite different from the sterility found in the modern, Western model and it's one of the reasons I so enjoy Africa!

This is something we can learn from the African community. As Westerners, we too can include our children more fully in the community. Instead of separating our children from the marketplace, putting them metaphorically by the side of the road and shielding them from the rough and tumble of life, we need to enlist them to be our co-journeyers in all that we do.

No longer are children in the streets of our neighborhoods. Because we live in fear, we shut up our children behind high fences that look more suited to be prisons than schools or preschools. I sometimes look at old photos of New York City from the late nineteenth century. Her streets were filled with children playing stickball while others sat watching on brownstone steps.

Whatever happened to that life?

When I was a young boy, I was given amazing freedom to ride my bike through the neighborhood and play football and baseball with friends in the streets. It was a different era, and I, along with many of my generation, lament the loss of that freedom for our children and our grandchildren.

Community Is Key

So learn a thing or two from the African way of life, hearken back to the New York City days, and include your children in your community, whatever it was before they came on the scene. You will find that your child adds a freshness to your community, and you'll also find that she will be welcomed by your friends and all who meet her.

Ubuntu: I Am Because You Are

The African concept of *ubuntu* refers to the interconnectedness of all human beings: we are all part of a greater community; we cannot succeed without the help of others, and they cannot succeed without us. Loosely translated, the word *ubuntu* means, "I am because you are": only together can we prosper.

4. The Cornerstone of Health

Last, but not least, parents are called to care for their child's health. To accomplish this goal, there are three steps you must take.

A. Find a Pediatrician

Babies are frail and vulnerable creatures. They need a team of people to look after them and care for them. Pediatricians, along with family and friends, are part of the team parents engage to help in the task.

So an early task parents must accomplish is to find a pediatrician to share with them in caring for their babies' health. Pediatricians bring medical experience, comfort, and advice and make the first months and years with baby safer and more secure.

How to Choose a Pediatrician

There are many important questions new parents should ask when looking for a doctor to care for their babies. Here's my list:

- Where did they do their training? Pediatricians who train in excellent teaching programs learn from the best teachers. They have a solid foundation and carry this forward into their careers.
- Are they board certified? Board certification is not a requirement to practice, but it means those doctors are committed to the profession and, after their formal training, took the time and effort to pass rigorous examinations.
- Are they currently affiliated with a teaching hospital? Doctors who teach are, by definition, still learning. This usually means that they are also up to date in their knowledge base and current in their skills.

- Are they readily accessible? Doctors who don't return phone calls and who have very limited office hours will not be available to you when you need them.
- Do they come highly recommended? The individuals who know doctors better than anyone else are the nurses at your local hospital. They work with them on a daily basis and know who the strong doctors are. Call the charge nurse in your local nursery and the charge nurse in labor and delivery. Ask for three names from both. Frequently, there will be a name (or names) that pops up more than once. Call these physicians and schedule interviews with them. After your interviews, you will know which doctor and which office fits your needs.

B. Get Your Children Vaccinated

Vaccinations are foundational for the health of your baby and are a big part of the medical care for children during their first year. There are more vaccines now than ever, and this can be overwhelming and confusing to parents, but get on board and get the job done. Have your pediatrician explain the various immunizations, why they are given, and what side effects you can expect after shots are given.

Making the Hurt of Vaccinations Go Away

Researchers have found that babies who breastfeed while they are receiving their immunizations cried for an average of thirty-eight seconds less and had lower pain scores compared to children who were not breastfed during vaccinations. In fact, breastfeeding was more effective in reducing vaccine pain than maternal cuddling, massage, pain creams, injection site sprays, and sugar water.

Pediatricians give vaccines to young babies because it is during the early months of life that children are most vulnerable to infection. Newborns don't have immature immune systems, necessarily, it's just that their immune systems are "naive." In other words, they haven't lived long enough to encounter and conquer the many viruses that are coming their way. As one author put it, the immune systems of newborns need "tutoring." Immunizations are the teachers your baby's immune system needs.

Influenza in an infant, for example, is a potentially life-threatening illness. In a fourteen-year-old individual, influenza is also a serious infection, but rarely is it life threatening. By the time someone is fourteen, his immune system has encountered influenza germs and learned to fight the infection off and/or protect his body from serious harm. A baby's body can't do this because it hasn't learned how to yet. Vaccines teach babies' bodies how to protect themselves, so giving vaccinations during your child's first year protects her from infections that can have profound ramifications due to her youth.

Children are in the pediatric office more frequently during the first year, which provides a convenient opportunity to receive vaccines, especially the ones that require multiple boosters.

Needles Galore

I recently had a mother in my practice who decided to defer vaccinations for her daughter until she was two years of age. I told her from the start this was not a good idea. First, her daughter was missing out on the value of vaccinations during a time in her life when she was most vulnerable to serious infections. Second, giving immunizations to two-year-old children is a challenge. By this age, children are very perceptive. They know exactly what doctors' offices are all about, and—do I need to state this?—two-year-old children abhor getting shots!

So at two years of age, this little girl was going to have a lot of making up to do.

As her daughter approached two, however, this mommy learned some unfortunate news. The exclusive preschool that she desperately wanted her daughter to attend would accept her for the fall session only with the proviso that the child be fully vaccinated by the time the term began.

For Mom, it was panic time. And for the child, it became a different kind of panic time! What I had failed to accomplish after two years of cajoling, the fancy preschool down the street got done in one afternoon. But that poor little girl!

We had to double up on all her missed vaccinations to get her caught up. Needless to say, this wasn't a pleasant task.

VACCINES WORK

The technology that has been developed after years of painstaking research has yielded a crop of vaccines that have changed the world. Children are healthier today than ever before. Infant mortality has plunged over the past century, and common illnesses like chicken pox, which once circulated perpetually through the community, are nearly gone. Viruses like polio, which left paralyzed boys and girls in its wake, have been vanquished from entire continents. Bacteria like *N. meningitidis*, which took limbs and lives, have been quelled.

Such is the power of vaccinations.

Consider the innovation that has gone into cell phones. The technological revolution that allows us to now carry sophisticated computers in our pockets has occurred in the medical field as well. Does anyone really want to return to rotary phones? From MRIs to new antiviral medicines to vaccinations, medicine has advanced over the past fifty years at the same pace that your telephone has. Put this innovation to work for you and your family.

Vaccinations Are for Those Who Care for Your Baby Too

Those who care for your newborn baby, like grandmothers and nannies, should also be vaccinated, particularly with an annual flu immunization and the Tdap vaccine, which prevents older individuals from passing whooping cough to young babies.

C. Attend a CPR and First-Aid Course

One evening, Leslie and I were having dinner with friends at a neighborhood restaurant. While enjoying a lively conversation, I happened to look over to a table close to ours and notice an older man who seemed to be choking on his food. I immediately went over to him and confirmed my observation. Grabbing him from behind, I performed the Heimlich maneuver, and a piece of unchewed beef popped out of his mouth. It was a dramatic moment that was over as quickly as it began.

The man, clearly terrified and embarrassed all at the same time, put his head on the table and caught his breath. I walked back to my seat, shaken, but thankful for knowing how to save his life.

One of the best investments that families can make is readiness when it comes to simple first aid and CPR for their children. The hope is you will never have to use your knowledge, but things happen, always in the moments we least expect, and when they do, a quick response is required.

As a parent, you're often the first responder when emergencies happen. It is wise to be ready. CPR and first-aid training should *not* be considered an option but an obligation and investment to your child's health. Do it before you need it. Classes are available from your local Red Cross or local hospital.

The Family You Build

You are building something very special with your family. Your faith, your parenting style, the community you engage your child in, and the health of your child are all cornerstones that new parents need to build upon.

What you are constructing is bigger and more complicated and more wondrous than you realize when you start, and it will endure long after you are gone. Therefore, build with intention. Build upon secure foundations, and build with common sense. Great families that are constructed well are a glory to behold and bring delight and blessings for generations.

7

The Wonders of the First (Maniacal) Year

SURPRISE: There's an electrical storm going on inside your baby's head.

A newborn infant is born with one hundred billion nerve cells in her brain! This is roughly equivalent to the number of stars that are in the Milky Way galaxy, and this vast array of neurons is *ready for action.*

At birth, your baby's neurons haven't yet made all the vital interconnections with one another that will allow them to work in synchrony, so when a baby is born, a chaotic, helter-skelter, messy race begins. Neurophysiologists call it *neuronal blooming,* and it happens at a breathtaking pace.

Think of it like this: You're at a party with one hundred billion of your closest friends who all know each other but who haven't seen each other for some time. It's a wild happening! The place is insanely loud and raucous. People are shouting across the room to

each other, laughing, embracing, and excitedly sharing phone numbers and email addresses.

These are the fireworks that are going on (*and keep going on*)
within the small space of your newborn baby's cranium.

In the brain, neuronal blooming happens when *axons* (the send-
ers of nerve impulses) and *dendrites* (the receivers of nerve impulses) contact one another and form *synapses*. This is how young
"pollywog" neurons start talking to one another, how the wiring of
the brain forms, and how information begins to flow. Babies' brains
are approximately one-quarter the size of an adult's brain, and the
growth that occurs in the size of the brain, from baby to adult, is
due to the interconnections, called *white matter*, that are being
made during these early years of life.

Everything that happens to a child during the first few months
of life causes more connections to form. Babies are "digitalizing"
everything they experience. When Auntie Sarah massages the
legs of her newborn niece Emery, new synapses are made. When
baby Luli goes to the park and feels the wind fluff her hair, new
synapses are formed. And the more any one event happens, the
more hardwired and enduring these connections become.

The Lights Go On

During your baby's first year of life, this relentless neuronal activity
goes on day in and day out, moment by moment. Early on in brain
development, more than one million new synaptic connections are
forming *every second!* Ultimately, more than *one quadrillion* connections will be made during the first few years of life. This is an astronomical number that is difficult to comprehend, even with the
billions of neurons we have at our disposal!

But early on, in the race to connect, the fecund young brain
overreaches and makes more connections than it really needs. A

two-year-old child has *twice* as many neuronal synapses as an adult before pruning begins. Continuously used pathways are maintained and strengthened, while those tenuous, unused connections are degraded and lost.

During the first year, however, your baby's brain is in the flush of neuronal blooming. And although parents are not able to see the explosive electric light parade going on in their babies' brains, they see it played out in everyday life through the relentless developmental changes that their babies achieve.

It's analogous to looking out across a giant metropolis at dusk from a mountaintop. As darkness crowds in on the landscape, the tall buildings illuminate as the people in them turn on the lights. Streetlights flicker, drivers turn on their headlights, and the brilliance of the city spreads until the entire landscape is aglow.

This is what it's like to behold a newborn baby progress through the first year. Newborns barely have the neck strength to lift their heads; they sleep the majority of the day and ingest only milk, and their only utterances are a cry. At one year of age—a mere 365 days later—your child is learning to walk, says a word or two, and eats a full diet. He is an insatiably curious toddler who drinks everything in as his nervous system continues to come online.

Parents will tell you that they can literally see new changes happen daily. Ask any father or mother, when they come back from even a short business trip, if their children look different to them upon their return. Their answer is always a firm *yes!*

Oh, and lest I forget to mention it, these adorable, toddling, curious little one-year-old creatures have also developed personalities.

Warning: Guard Yourself Against "Milestone Anxiety"

Every child is different, and every stage of your daughter's or son's development won't parallel that of any other child, so beware. Employ *great* caution when you compare your baby to other babies. I know this is a near-impossible recommendation to follow because it goes against the grain of our human nature, but constantly measuring your child to other children will only create anxiety for you. As children grow and mature, parents realize that the majority of our hand-wringing was unnecessary vexation.

I spend much of my day discussing normal developmental milestones with parents, and I find that nearly all parents have, at times, concerns and worries about their children when it comes to growth and development. This is the nature of parenthood.

That said, the following developmental stages that we are about to discuss are *generalities.* They will not exactly reflect the progress of your child—*or any other given child*, for that matter—because every child is different, and *no* individual is generic.

Finally, if you have ongoing concerns regarding any aspect of your child's development, these are issues that should be discussed with your pediatrician.

Beyond the First Month of Life

We have discussed the wonder of a baby's first dynamic month of life in chapter 3, but after those first four weeks, new development, equally wonderful, continues to occur with your child. Those drowsy, somnolent babies begin to come alive and engage the world around them.

Parents who have spent the first month "bailing water" without much positive reinforcement from their baby finally get some hard-earned and well-deserved rewards. Those early smirks turn into smiles, and those faint, dove-like coos, happy murmurs, and throaty growls become proto-conversations. These are some of the beautiful little moments and miracles parents will appreciate during their babies' second month of life. This is also the month that babies start waking up and interacting with their world and the time that true, social smiles are seen. Throughout the first month, parents debate in their minds whether their infants' smirks were meant for them. Now those evanescent half smiles, often labeled by moms and dads as "gas grins," are replaced by clear social smiles that are, without doubt, the *real deal*.

In addition, babies, during month two, become interactive. When you smile at your baby, she beams back at you a broad smile. This is thrilling after a long, cold month of "baby hibernation." These back-and-forth communications with their mothers and fathers indicate that babies are beginning to take note of their parents and that a shared experience is occurring. For parents hungry for their children to respond to them, there is nothing in life more satisfying.

These mommy-daddy-baby exchanges often begin with a quiet coo. It's a hushed but satisfied sound that comes forth from your baby after she has been fed and changed. It's almost as if she's saying, "Great work, Mommy! I am totally satisfied!"

Visually, they track contrasting objects around the room and begin to open their mouths when presented with a breast or a bottle.

Motor-wise, babies' random movements become smoother, and they begin to unfist their hands more (about 50 percent of the time) and put them in their mouths. Finally, they will firmly grasp items that are placed into their hands.

Your Three-Month-Old Baby

By three months, your baby has completed the first quarter year of his life. Pediatrician, writer, and lecturer Harvey Karp, M.D., is one of those who designates these months as the *fourth trimester.* It's during this time that babies fully wake up and start checking things out. They have emerged from their primordial slough and begin to make peace with the world around them. They fuss less and are less irritable, and their colicky tummy issues are generally behind them.

Three months also seems to be the age when babies realize that they are *one of us.* I joke with parents that at three months, they finally decide to forgive their mothers for giving birth to them and stop their whining about wanting to get back into the womb. When this happens, they turn into sweet little babies who are utterly delicious, guileless, innocent, and ready to flirt with those around them. As Alison Gopnik and her coauthors write in their book *The Scientist in the Crib: Minds, Brains, and How Children Learn,* three-month-old children engage in "an intricate dance, a kind of wordless conversation, a silly love song, pillow talk [that] is sheer heaven." This all starts at three months of age.

The Best Age

I am sometimes asked my opinion about what age is the "best age." If I had to choose a moment in the life of a child that I find most wonderful and precious, this is it! Three-month-old children are my favorites! They are sweet little people with wide-open eyes and a ready smile for all those who look in their direction.

By three months, moms are also finally getting more rest and are beginning to feel more like they are getting control of their lives again. Most mothers have also guided their children into a more reasonable and predictable schedule. These factors add to the pleasantness of the age.

Physically speaking, three-month-old babies prop themselves up at a forty-five-degree angle and begin rolling to their sides. They bring their hands to their mouths and begin to primitively bat at objects. Their little hands are still fisted half of the time, but they are intentionally opening them more and continue to grasp items that are placed into their hands.

Parents will also notice that their babies are becoming more vocal, with louder chortles and excited and happy verbal responses to caretakers when they are spoken to.

Your Four-Month-Old Baby

Four-month-old babies begin what I call the "touch all" stage of life, with improved eye-hand coordination and an understanding of how far objects are away from them. They're also very alert and very chatty!

This is the time when a handful of developmental events come online. First, babies who have been strengthening their backs and core muscles during their tummy time workouts will begin to turn their heads and roll. Their first roll is usually from stomach to back. It's the baby version of tuck and roll.

By four months, babies have been batting with their hands for several weeks, but up until now, these have been random movements. Now babies begin to employ true, purposeful reaching. Four-month-old babies keep their hands open nearly all the time, and those hands are creatively at work exploring the world.

Beware: Your Baby Is a Rolling Risk

At four months of age, babies constitute what I call a *rolling risk*. If you leave your young one alone on a changing table or a couch or a bed, even a split second, he'll find a way to tumble off it.

I have taken many a telephone call from crying or chagrined parents whose children have done this very thing. One of my patients, *on his first roll ever*, toppled off a three-foot-tall table, landed squarely on his head on a hardwood floor, and fractured his skull. All ultimately turned out well and good for this little fellow in the end, but it was a tough beginning to his rolling career.

Babies this age love to grasp, grab, reach, and pull on *everything*, especially their mothers' hair.

One of our children's favorite tricks at this age is what I call the *tablecloth pull*. I've had whole plates of food tumble into my lap while trying to eat with one of my children on my knee. And watch out if you dare to take this tiny, destructive creature to the supermarket. If you get too close to the cereal shelves, you'll end up with a pile of Cheerios boxes on the floor. And when the crashing is over, your child will show no remorse. Instead, she'll smile with glee as she realizes that she now possesses the power to cause great chaos.

Now is also the time that parents must exercise caution with hot and sharp items. Don't try to have a cup of hot tea or coffee with an ever-reaching four-month-old baby nearby. Accidents with hot and sharp objects can cause serious harm to your baby.

Since four months is the time babies get creative with their hands, this is the perfect time to give a baby a rattle. They're learning how to hold things, and making noise while grasping an object is an added bonus. Rattles fit these developmental drives and their little palms perfectly.

Socially, four-month-old babies laugh aloud, get excited when they see people, and love to have back-and-forth conversations. In fact, at four months, babies *love* the company of others and become more playful with them. When the playing ends, they'll often cry for more.

Gross motor–wise, your four-month-old daughter now has enough leg strength to support her trunk well. She'll love to do this, and despite what some people say, allowing your baby girl to bear her weight *will not* cause her legs to bow. Her upper body strength is also increasing, so when she is pulled with her arms into a sitting position, she no longer has head lag. During tummy time, babies push up to nearly a ninety-degree angle.

Four months is likewise the period when children begin the early stages of teething; however, the actual appearance of teeth is still a way off. Teeth (usually the two bottom teeth) erupt between six and seven months of age, but the teething period precedes eruption by several months. You will know teething is beginning when your baby begins to drool profusely and chew on everything he can find.

Chew toys are also great to introduce now. They're helpful to mitigate some of the pain of teething and also assuage a child's insatiable need to chew. Better a chew toy than a daddy's finger . . . or a mommy's nipple!

SURPRISE: The Truth About Teething

There is a lot of debate about what symptoms—other than drooling and chewing—teething causes. It is my observation that teething can cause some changes in bowel patterns (like diarrhea and color changes to the stool), but it is also my experience that *teething does not cause fever.*

Along with four-month teething comes *tasting*. Right about now, parents will notice that nearly everything will go into the mouths of their babies. This can be a very distressing time because some of the things your child will put in their mouths will utterly disgust you. But this is how our children discover the world in which they live, and this is yet another reason God gave babies parents.

Finally, four months is the age when parents need to be more proactive in setting schedules for their children. For many families, these routines have been evolving over the past couple of months already. Parents will be pleased to note that their children naturally fall into and happily acquiesce to a more predictable schedule.

Your Five-Month-Old Baby

By five months, babies are beginning to roll from their backs to their stomachs, which requires new, different, and more challenging skills for an infant. They begin to sit, with pelvic support, in a tripod position, leaning forward with their hands on the floor. They are now fully capable of grasping objects with their hands in a primitive fashion. We call this a *palmar grasp*. They hold their hands together and transfer objects from one hand, to mouth, to the other hand. They still mouth everything they grasp, in a continuation of the teething that started the previous month.

Around this time, you might notice your baby persistently tugging at her ears. While your first thought may be that she has an ear infection, it is more than likely just another display of her discovering her world—and that includes her own body. Fingers, toes, and any other protruding parts are ripe for exploration. Unless she is obviously in discomfort, with crying, a fever, food refusal, or fussiness, you can categorize this behavior as blossoming curiosity.

Socially, five-month-old babies show clear signs of bonding with their parents and caregivers. They are beginning to express emotion with sounds other than cries to let you know when they are happy, angry, or bored and even their likes and dislikes. Verbally, five-month-old babies are beginning to babble vowel sounds like *aah*, *eeh*, and *oooh*. And they finally begin to laugh at all those silly faces you are making!

Your Six-Month-Old Baby

Six months into the journey of parenting, moms and dads will be absolutely astounded how much their babies have changed. A six-month-old infant is a much more sophisticated baby than he was way back in his first month of life.

By six months, babies are very social, full of smiles, and truly delightful in all ways. They enjoy mirrors, often touching their reflections in the mirror and vocalizing. They are beginning to jabber with repetitive use of consonants and vowels like *ba-ba-ba*, *da-da-da*, and *mi-mi-mi*. They will stop momentarily to verbal commands of *no* and are beginning to develop early signs of stranger anxiety. They clearly know new faces and may be ill at ease with people they don't know.

SURPRISE: Stranger anxiety means your baby is bonding with you!

Stranger Anxiety

Between six and nine months, your baby will begin to demonstrate anxiety and will shy away from new people in his environment. This can be baffling and sometimes embarrassing to parents because, up until now, their child was amicable with strangers and coopera-tive when he was picked up and cared for by new individuals.

Although this change may surprise parents because a "new" person sometimes is a beloved aunt, uncle, or even a grandparent, the intensity of your baby's anxiety is a function of his attachment to his mom and dad.

Therefore, parents should look at stranger anxiety as *good* because it indicates that their children see them as their trusted foundation.

Physically, six-month-old babies can pivot around when they are in an upright, seated position and can bear weight on one hand. Their core strength is increasing, which means they can roll easily, but they usually prefer to play in an upright position instead of lying down while awake. When it comes to fine-motor skills, six-month-old babies transfer objects easily from hand to hand, feed themselves and hold their bottles.

This is the time when I start imploring patients to childproof their homes. Untethered, six-month-old children are my definition of *trouble*, which is why I generally tell parents (tongue in cheek) that now's the time to break out the barbed wire! This is the age when babies begin to explore their world, and they do this unceas-ingly. With their new abilities to pivot and roll, they can cover great distances in the blink of an eye!

Six months of age is also the time when I like to begin solid foods. Your child has been watching you eat for a couple of months now, and she will often reach out and try to grab any foods that are within her range. Now it's time to indulge her curiosity.

Introducing Solid Foods

Q: When should I start feeding solids to my baby?

A: Children all over the world are fed differently, but there are a few overriding recommendations that pediatricians make in the Western world:

- We generally suggest that babies be breastfed for *at least* the first six months of life. I encourage new mothers to give their babies nothing but breast milk for the first six months unless the mother has a limited milk supply and needs to supplement with formula or donated breast milk.
- At six months, I recommend introducing the first solids to your baby, starting with soft and nutritious foods that are easy to digest. (See chapter 8.)

Q: Can I give food to my baby before he is six months old?

A: Even if your baby seems interested in food before he is six months old, it is important that you don't introduce food to him too early. Babies younger than six months have a virginal gut that is still maturing.

That said, there are times when I *do* allow babies to begin feeding beginning as early as four months of age. It is not my go-to recommendation, but there are some children who are large for their age, are waking frequently at night to feed, and simply need extra calories.

Q: What if my baby doesn't swallow food yet or isn't even interested in solids?

A: While some babies are excited to try new foods at six months, not all babies share that interest! It is not unusual for babies to take longer than six months before they finally have a desire to eat solid foods. Be patient with your child, and don't force it, but continue to offer food to him periodically. It might take a while, but he will get it!

Q: What are the best "first foods" I can give to my baby?

A: Choose foods that are nutritious and soft, like avocados, sweet potatoes (cooked and cut into small pieces, or puréed), bananas, strawberries, mango, peas, and sugar-free all-natural applesauce.

Cereals (rice, oats, barley, and quinoa) have been the starter foods for generations, and despite recent criticism of their nutritional value, I still believe cereals have their place and continue to recommend them to parents routinely. However, due to recent reports of higher-than-allowed arsenic levels in commercially available rice cereals, I now recommend that parents avoid this grain until further notice.

Your Seven-Month-Old Baby

By seven months of age, babies have been reconfigured into delightful, bubbly little packages. They love to bear weight when they are held in your arms and bounce up and down in this position. This is also the age when they become more aware of music and frequently will rock and sway their bodies to the beat.

Physically, they are mastering control of their core strength, and they are now able to sit without support, arms at their sides. The latest addition to their fine-motor skill set is called the *radialpalmar grasp,* which means that they grasp objects using the sides of their hands.

At seven months, babies are beginning to understand cause and effect. They let go of something and it falls to the ground. This is fascinating to them, and they will do it many times over again!

When it comes to speech, seven-month-olds increase the variety of consonants in their babbling, and their sheer amount (and volume!) of babbling increases greatly too. They show greater verbal understanding, looking at familiar objects when they are named.

Socially, they indicate their desires by looking from object to parent and back again when they want something.

Your Eight-Month-Old Baby

By eight months, babies are now able to get into a sitting position without help. They scoot across the floor in an army crawl and are beginning to pull themselves up to a kneeling position. When it comes to fine-motor skills, your eight-month-old baby will bang a spoon and employ a *scissor grasp*, which means grabbing objects with all four fingers and the side of the thumb. They take cubes out of a cup and pull pegs out of holes. They're also able to pick up finger foods like small pieces of fruit or crackers with their fingertips.

One of the biggest milestones that occurs around this time is the development of what is called *object permanence*. Your baby will begin looking for an object when it has fallen from a high chair, for example, and she will anticipate that your face will reappear in a game of peekaboo.

Visually, your eight-month-old baby will follow the gaze of others, looking toward the objects or people their caregivers look at.

Verbally, they begin to have non-reduplicate babble. In other words, rather than babbling *ma-ma-ma-ma* or *da-da-da-da*, they will begin to say words like *ma-ma* or *da-da*—though it will take another couple of months before they associate meaning with these words.

Your Nine-Month-Old Baby

By nine months of age, babies are making great advances. Gross motor–wise, they're able to crawl very well on their knees and crawl in a bearlike fashion on their hands and feet. Some children this age are also beginning to pull themselves up to stand on couches and chairs.

Fine motor–wise, they have matured to a *radial-digital* grasp, which means they can grasp items with two fingers (the index and middle finger) and their thumbs. They enjoy banging two blocks together and smoothly pass blocks from one hand to the other.

Cognitively, nine-month-old babies are beginning to study objects more carefully and understand cause and effect. They ring bells after being shown how to do so and drag out-of-reach toys to themselves with a string.

Socially, they continue to experience stranger anxiety and become clingy with their caretakers when they sense fear. They also now recognize and orient when their names are spoken.

Verbally, they begin to imitate sounds and continue their development of non-reduplicate babbling sounds. Anyone who has spent time with nine-month-old babies will tell you that they are veritable noise machines.

Your Ten-Month-Old Baby

For those who neglected my earlier childproofing advice, it is now time to quickly childproof your house! By the tenth month, most babies are crawling well around the house, and they're fast. They are also able to sidle along furniture while holding on with two hands. We call this *cruising*. They're also able to stand while holding on with one hand and walk when parents hold both of their hands.

Fine motor–wise, they have matured in their grasping abilities. They now employ an *inferior pincer grasp*, grasping objects with the thumb and the side of the index finger. They clumsily release a cube held in their hands and can now isolate the index finger and point at objects. This is the age too when they are beginning to drink from a cup.

Ten-month-old babies fully understand object permanence and uncover toys that are placed under cloths. They love to play peek-aboo and begin to wave bye-bye to people. Emotionally and socially, they experience fear, and they look immediately when their names are called.

Verbally, they are beginning to specifically say words like *dada* and *mama*, which comes as a pure delight to parents.

Your Eleventh-Month-Old Baby

By eleven months of age, infants begin to point at objects for others to see as well. This is an important social tool for infants. Such gestures represent a prelinguistic way to get parents to retrieve an object for them.

In the realm of gross-motor skills, an eleven-month-old baby has advanced to the point where he can walk with only one hand held and cruise along furniture with ease, using just one hand to stabilize himself. He is also experimenting with early standing, which lasts only momentarily. Fine motor–wise, eleven-month-olds can stir with a spoon, throw objects, and when being dressed, they (finally!) begin to cooperate with their arms and legs.

By eleven months, babies' love for music, which began several months earlier, blooms. They bounce along to the beat, and verbally, they're even beginning to vocalize some of the lyrics.

Cognitively, they can find objects that are hidden under cups, and they look at pictures in books in a sustained way. Socially, they give objects back to adults and indicate when they need help from adults. They might even stop an activity when they are told *no*.

Your Baby's First Words

What will be your baby's first word? I like to ask my patients' parents what their children's first words were, and I get great array of answers, including *bubbles*, *macho*, and the name of their dog. The first word one of our daughters spoke was *agua*, an interesting choice since neither my wife nor I speak Spanish in the home.

Your One-Year-Old Baby

By the time your baby is one year old, she is radically different from the newborn you brought home from the hospital, and you will marvel at the changes that have occurred in the past twelve months.

One-year-olds are curious beyond belief, and this will only increase in their second year of life. They babble nonstop and even utter a word or two that has true meaning like *mama* or *dada*. They are very sophisticated in assessing items and even the feelings of their caretakers. They point to objects and anticipate that you, the adult in the room, will share an interest in the object that they are pointing to. Your one-year-old also knows that if someone else is pointing at an object, she too should look in that direction.

Furthermore, by one year of age, the entire universe becomes something within their reach. One-year-old children are interested in *everything, all the time*. If parents have not childproofed their homes by now, they are in serious trouble. Your little foraging bear is going to ravage the place, and he won't think twice about destroying even the most valuable of objects.

It will not come as a surprise that babies this age also have excellent memories and communicate very effectively without using words. They like to shake, throw, and bang objects. They find objects that are hidden, copy gestures, play "in and out" games, and can even follow simple directions like, "Get the toy."

For fine-motor skills, they can now scribble after being shown what to do. They demonstrate a *fine pincer grasp*, reaching and grasping objects with the index finger and the thumb from above. They are also beginning to stack blocks on top of each other, making towers of two blocks or more. One-year-olds are even more co-operative now in dressing, and they're able to finger-feed themselves very well. They take hats off and lift lids off boxes to find toys.

Gross motor–wise, one-year-old children get into a sitting position without help, pull to a stand, and stand alone, and many are beginning to take their first steps.

One-year-old children have arrived. They have made gigantic progress in acquiring skills. Watching a child—*your own* child—grow from a frail infant to a solid and sturdy one-year-old is nothing short of watching, up close and personal, the unfolding of a perfectly choreographed, unmitigated miracle.

A Whirlwind of Miracles

The first year is perhaps the most dynamic year of human life; a whirlwind of changes, it's a year filled with wonder. The tender rosebud you brought home from the hospital has bloomed into radiant color, and you were a witness to all the action.

The tiny baby, whom you now barely remember, has awakened and grown into a big boy or girl. Looking at the world as a fresh and exciting place to be, your son or daughter has begun *his or her own* journey in life. It's impossible to be around your child without feeling a sense of accomplishment and quest.

Finally, the ultimate gift that children bring is laughter. Their eyes aglow with infectious exuberance, babies make us laugh.

There is never a day that goes by that I don't find myself laughing with the parents of the children that I care for. It's a happy laugh.

And with our mirth, there is also great hope. Such are the gifts that children give.

8

. . . . .

Establishing Healthy Patterns
in the First Year

Newborn babies are utterly dependent, fledgling chicks. At birth, babies do next to nothing. They don't smile, they can't lift their heads or turn over, and they require constant care. One-year-old babies are quite different. By one year of age, children are on the threshold of walking. They reach for and manipulate items with excellent dexterity; they babble unceasingly and appear to understand every word their parents say. These insatiable and feverishly curious blurs of humanity look and act nothing like their former fragile, primordial, newborn selves.

For parents, witnessing this marvelous transformation, visible changes happen daily. But parents aren't just passive witnesses to the process; they play an active and, in my opinion, a *determining role* in how their children will mature and develop during the remarkable and miraculous first 365 days of life.

You're in Charge

But there's one concept parents must grasp from the moment their children are born: *the parents are in charge.* In the context of your family, you're the ones calling the shots.

Some people have difficulty with the concept of power differentials, even when it comes to their children. Hierarchy, for some, induces stress. I contend, however, that everywhere in life and in your community, from the grocery store to the airport to your child's elementary school, there are those whose *job* it is to be in charge. Police officers are granted the authority to compel you to follow traffic laws. School principals have the authority to discipline unruly students.

In the context of a family, someone must assume authority—*and newborn babies are not ready for the job.*

Your baby, even from an early age, will do his best to usurp your authority, but he is both unformed and uninformed. I'm not being unkind; I just know kids. They need to learn from and follow people who *do* know what's going on. This is the job moms and dads must perform. The parents' role is one of leadership and guidance. It's our solemn responsibility to perform it to the best of our abilities.

> *Babies are not born resilient; [but] they are born malleable.*
> —ALLAN SCHORE

Reining in the Wild Child

The first year is without a doubt the most dynamic year in the life of a human being. No other time in life compares to the radical changes that occur in growth and development, so this is the year parents will find themselves busy establishing schedules, setting limits, and reining in this nascent little human.

The three behavior milestones that parents need to consider and focus on during baby's first year are:

- **Establishing predictable schedules**, including playtime, nap time, bath time, and downtime.

- **Getting your baby to sleep through the night.**
- **Starting your baby on solid food.**

All Humans Look for Patterns

My grandson Bennett loves to have a book read to him before bedtime. Recently, my wife and I were babysitting him in our home, and we attempted to put him down to bed *without* reading to him. He immediately rebelled. It took a moment or two for us to realize that we had forgotten this important prequel to his bedtime, but then we snuggled up together and read him a book or two. When we finished, Bennett's universe was restored to order, and he was ready to cooperate. He then went down in his crib without a peep and with a smile on his face.

Even from the very start, human babies look for rhythms and patterns. As a general concept, consistency and predictability are important when it comes to raising children. They're born ready and eager to etch structure into their days and enjoy anticipating what's next on any given day's agenda. That said, there is no reason to strictly adhere to a rigid schedule that disallows all freedoms. Getting your son down at eight rather than seven is okay if you want to take him with you for dinner with friends. Children adjust well to these minor schedule variations without harm.

But developing patterns of living that your child will inherently understand is an important part of healthy parenting during the first year. Your sons and daughters will derive comfort from the rhythms of life, and these patterns can be established much earlier than most people realize.

But children need to be guided and taught how to live life. They're born willing, but they need moms and dads who are prepared to take the time to teach and instill these patterns into their lives. This takes work and a commitment to molding and disciplining your child.

The Need for Direction

Jean-Jacques Rousseau was an eighteenth-century philosopher and writer whose work influenced the Enlightenment in France and later, after his death, the French Revolution. Rousseau wrote extensively about children and looked at them as a prototype for his theory of the "noble savage," a theory that proposed that there existed, in the primitive world, naturally noble individuals who knew truth and lived accordingly. According to him, it was modernity that corrupted mankind, especially competitive capitalism. In Rousseau's words, "Man's breath is fatal to his fellow men."

Extrapolating these kind thoughts of the noble savage to the nature of children, Rousseau proposed that children are naturally born knowing right from wrong, and given the opportunity to choose, they will choose the right thing to do.

Unfortunately, he got it all wrong! If Rousseau had actually *raised* children, rather than abandoning to the state the children he fathered with his mistress, Thérèse Levasseur, he would have known better. The truth is the polar opposite. Although children are the cutest and most delightful little creatures imaginable, they are gripped with all the guile and self-centeredness that comes with being a human. When they are very young, they just don't have the wherewithal to manifest these naughty, innate, human qualities. But they will. So children will need your parental guidance and direction, even from their earliest days.

Guiding Our Children Through Life

The biblical book of Proverbs is filled with old wisdom. There it is written, "Discipline your children, and they will give you peace; they will bring you the delights you desire." The ancients were not a bunch of stodgy old men who wanted to throw water on the party. They were wise individuals who studied human nature and came to conclusions about what constituted "good living." When it came to guiding and raising their children, there was no confusion. They understood that discipline was an absolute necessity during the early years of life—and they also understood the rewards that later come when parents impose *their will* on their children.

I know this sounds a bit regressive in today's permissive and freewheeling climate, but children who are left to themselves don't do well. Dads and moms who leave it to chance or are overly lenient with their children raise unpleasant, ungrateful, and whiny kids. Parents of these children end up spending their lives begging and lecturing them endlessly. When they are called to explain to teachers and others in authority why their children are such ill-behaved malcontents, they're left feeling embarrassed, speechless, and powerless to do anything about it.

On the other hand, mothers and fathers who make guidance a priority, though it is often unpleasant work, enjoy tangible benefits for their efforts.

Writer and physician Leonard Sax, M.D., put it this way: "Self-control is not innate." In his book *The Collapse of Parenting*, he wrote, "No child is born knowing the rules." This is certainly true, and this becomes very evident during the second year of life, but it is equally true in the first year of life as well.

Gentle admonitions are necessary for all children. They yield a secure and delightful son or daughter. Guidance should be applied to all behaviors, from sitting in a car seat (an essential thing to do) to biting your best friend (not a good thing to do).

On Never Saying *No*

I have cared for a few families over my career who have decided to never use the word *no* with their children. When they share this decision with me, I am always utterly flabbergasted. "How can this be possible?" I ask. Their response typically goes along this line: "We only want our child to hear and know positive words and thoughts in our home."

These are lofty goals, but these parents, like Rousseau, have missed the mark. Author and family psychologist John Rosemond calls the word *no* vitamin N and says that it's the "essential vitamin we have never heard of." However, this vitamin, asserts Rosemond, is probably more important to your child's development than all other vitamins combined. I can't agree more. Children who suffer from vitamin N deficiency become, as Rosemond puts it, "sullen and ungrateful" individuals. Author and University of Toronto professor Jordan B. Peterson says it like this in his book *12 Rules for Life:* "Don't let your children do anything that makes you dislike them."

Our job as parents is to prepare our children for the world outside of the protected womb of our homes. Excluding the word *no* from your vocabulary with your children is a fairy-tale approach to parenting that borders on silliness. This is not how life operates, and these parents are preparing their children for a lifetime of frustration. When I look out my office window, I can see a vast sea of nos. No Parking, No Trespassing, and No Soliciting signs are everywhere.

The real world, the one that our children will ultimately enter, is filled with rules and regulations. We have a responsibility to both our children and our communities to prepare our children for the real world.

And believe it or not, getting them ready for that world starts in the first year. Step one is guiding your sons and daughters to a healthy schedule.

1. Getting Your Baby into the Groove

My patients often ask me in the first couple of weeks, "When should we begin to schedule our baby?" My answer is always nuanced. The truth is, when parents first get home with their babies, they're reeling. Before parents start scheduling their children, they first need to *survive!* Let's be honest: moms get beat up by the birthing process, even young women who are the fittest of the fit. Nobody skates through childbirth without some scars. And dads, while not having to deal with the physical trauma of childbirth, play an integral supportive role for the mother, so it's not a cakewalk for dads either.

So these early challenging days are a time to adjust. Start by getting used to the new parent paradigm. Keep your head above water and care for your baby. When they wake up, hold them and snuggle. When they need to be changed, be there for them. When they cry for food, feed them on demand. This is what your heart will lead you to do, so follow its tug. The adage "You can't spoil a newborn" is true, *but during the first couple of weeks, try your best to do so!*

Fortunately, early on, babies sleep a lot. This early hibernation is a blessing to their mothers, who need to rest as well. Within two to three weeks, however, parents will notice that their babies are awake longer during the day and they are becoming more alert. The puffiness that babies have around their eyes as newborns diminishes, so they can open their eyes wider and look around more. They first find their mothers and fathers, and then they turn their attention to all that is around them.

Additionally, babies begin to sleep for longer stretches during the night. By three to four weeks of age, many babies are sleeping up to four hours at a stretch. If a mother can coincide her sleep time with her child's, she will welcome these four-hour stretches, because this is the amount of sleep adults require to experience REM sleep, a key to being restored and feeling rested in the morning.

Other than sleeping, babies during the first few weeks spend their time feeding. Since breastfeeding mothers are half of the dyad, this means that they are being called into duty every two to three hours. I am a believer in on-demand feeding during the first month, and this is tough work, but there are rewards. Feeding times are usually followed by brief but pleasant awake times for baby. Full and content, they spend a few fleeting minutes looking around, discovering their world. These are precious moments for a mommy, daddy, and baby to enjoy together.

For Those Not in the Groove

This is the natural rhythm of the first month. It's a current that most newborn children understand and adapt to happily, and it also represents the first steps to a healthy schedule. The early needs that babies have (feeding, changing, and sleeping) and the response of their parents to these needs represents *proto-scheduling.* Most of my patients find this groove quickly, often within two to three weeks after coming home from the hospital, but if your baby *doesn't* fall into a discernible pattern, gentle nudging may be necessary.

I look at it like this: each day is divided into two unique periods—

day and night. Humans are awake and eating during the day, and we sleep and *don't* eat during the night. Babies are humans. You need to tell them this and let them know that they too need to fall in line with the program. This is straightforward stuff, but sometimes your child may not have gotten that memo. In fact, some kids get it upside-down wrong. They're awake and feeding throughout the entire night, then sleep like angels and hardly feed during the day. They're like wild teenagers. They're sleeping all day because they're planning on partying all night. We call this *reverse cycling*.

If reverse cycling goes on for too long, you'll both be exhausted and unhappy. Since your baby needs functioning parents, it's better to conquer this dragon early on. It generally isn't that hard to do. It's a matter of keeping your baby up more during the day and encouraging him to sleep at night. Here's what to do to get your baby in the groove.

Dr. Bob's Tried-and-True Prescription for the Loving Nudge

- **Wake Your Baby Early from Naps:** The "eat, awake, and sleep" cycle is a recurring theme for babies for the first weeks of life. Overall, children are only awake during the day from sixty to ninety minutes at a time, so it's still fine and important for your nocturnal-tending baby to nap during the day. They need their naps and several of them, but don't let these sleep times be too lengthy. Naps longer than two to three hours are going to come back to bite you later that night, especially if they occur in the late afternoon or early evening. So nudge your baby awake after a couple of hours of daytime sleeping.

- **Bathe Your Baby During the Day:** Baths arouse babies, so use them to keep your baby awake. Some children are not all that fond of bathing, but over time nearly all babies learn to love their bath times, and they become an integral part of their schedules. Don't bathe your child more than once a day, however. Too much bathing dries out the natural oils of the skin, and just like adults, baby skin can become rough and rashy.
- **Take Your Baby Outside:** Fresh air and sunlight awaken people. The wind in your child's face and the outdoor noises will arouse her as well.
- **Feed Your Baby:** Feeding also stimulates babies, and if babies feed well during the day, they will be less needy for milk during the night hours. I tell parents to push feedings during the day as much as your child will tolerate.
- **Establish a Bedtime Routine:** This helps your child know that it is bedtime. Babies need a relaxed and quiet environment to get to sleep.

The Scaffolding Goes Up

So getting your baby into the pattern of daily living is one of the first things that new parents need to do. Scheduling is like the scaffolding that goes up around a building before construction begins. It isn't pretty, but you need to put it up before you can proceed.

Proper scheduling of your baby doesn't come without a price. It will require your thoughtful attention, diligence, discipline, and time. If parents have been living, up to this point in life, a carefree and—shall we say, just for fun—a more slapdash lifestyle, parenthood is going to rein you in. All to-be parents have heard this before, but it's indeed true. That said, I'm a big believer in children also learning to adjust to their parents, so parents don't have to lose all their spontaneity or joie de vivre. Moms and dads obviously also need to accommodate their children, and they will, especially during the first months after delivery.

2. At Five Months, It's Time to Get Your Baby to Sleep

During the first months after birth, I am not strict about babies sleeping through the night. They are growing fast and their tummies are small, which means they need to feed often, including one to two or even three nighttime feeds. It is not uncommon for breastfeeding babies, who tend to be "grazers," to feed eight to twelve times each day. This is normal, and parents shouldn't feel any pressure to alter these natural early rhythms.

But at five months of age, I change my tune. By this age, children have doubled their birth weight and average between fourteen and sixteen pounds. They have already begun to consolidate a modicum of scheduling into their daily feeding and sleeping routines, and are now ready to be enrolled into my Two-Step Sleep-Training Program. It's a simple scheme:

Step 1 begins at five months and involves getting your child to go to bed *alone*, in their own sleep area.

Step 2 comes later (six to seven months, when children have started eating solid foods) and involves getting them to sleep through the night without feeds.

There is an abundance of sleep-training methods out there that parents can use to accomplish this important milestone. All of them center around the consensus that babies, to learn how to go to sleep, will probably have to spend some time crying alone in their cribs.

My recommendations are not markedly dissimilar from those of most other pediatricians, but there are a couple of caveats that I discuss with moms and dads. First, before they engage in a sleep-training program, parents need to be clear about what lies ahead.

They must *really* want their children to sleep through the night. If parents aren't totally committed to this goal and know, in advance, that they're incapable of enduring their children's crying, these parents should hold off on embarking on my scheme. They'll only dig themselves deeper into a sleeping quagmire if they start and then stop my plan. My only comment to these parents is that sleep training later doesn't get any easier as the days and months pass by; the task only becomes more challenging. So before you decide to forgo proactive sleep training, consider this advice.

Second, if you choose to follow my plan, make sure your child is well. Babies who are not well should be attended to. This is not the time to sleep train them. When they are healthy again, begin the process.

Third, mark off three to five days on your calendar when the two of you are home and can dedicate yourselves to the process. Moms and dads should sleep-train their children together because it can be emotionally wrenching, and you will need each other for moral support. Sleep training isn't a one-night stand for most babies. Going to sleep is a learned response, and it takes a handful of days for them to get on board with the program.

Fourth, I am one of those pediatricians who believes that picking up a child between crying episodes is okay. Some sleep specialists will strongly disagree with this opinion, but I think it is natural for a mother to *want* to pick up and comfort her baby when the baby is crying. Denying a mother this innate proclivity and denying a child the reassurance and comfort that picking him up provides only adds stress to the process. I concede that picking babies up between each crying episode may tend to drag out the process somewhat, but I believe a more nuanced approach to sleep training is ultimately more agreeable for babies, mothers, and fathers too.

Finally, my sleep plan is something that I have concocted over the years working with children and their parents. It is a matter of style and preference. There is no gospel when it comes to teaching a baby how to sleep through the night; every baby learns differently. I recently asked a group of pediatric colleagues what they said when they gave young parents sleep-training advice, and *each one of them* had slightly different recommendations. So with this being put on the table, I humbly proffer my sleep-training method to my readers as an option. I present it as guidelines or a suggestion rather than a proclamation. As with many other things in the parenting realm, ultimately, you will have to find what works best for you and your baby.

Dr. Bob's Tried-and-True Two-Step Sleep-Training Method

STEP 1: Getting your baby to go to sleep *alone.*

1. First, set a time in the early to midevening for your child's bedtime.

2. Since bedtime rituals are important, before placing your daughter in her crib, parents should go through their usual bedtime routines. Bathe and feed her, change her, pray with her, sing to her, read to her, and hug and rock her tenderly. This all takes time. Trying to hastily put your baby to bed, which we sometimes try to do as parents, usually doesn't work so well. Putting a baby to bed is like landing a 747 jumbo jet—a long and steady descent is required for a smooth landing.

3. Institute *sleep associations* for your baby. When it is time for bed, turn down the lights and lower the volume of the radio. Swaddle your baby, turn on the white noise (if you have it), and provide a soft, breathable "lovie" for them to hold. These presleep crutches are not only helpful during the night; they also signal to your baby that it's time for bed.

Rev Up the White Noise

White noise machines, which produce soft, predictable, and comforting sounds like a mommy's swishing heartbeat, rainfall, or ocean waves, are useful to block unwelcome noises like dripping faucets or noises from a television in the next apartment. Parents find white noise, played at low volume, is beneficial in calming their babies at bedtime and throughout the night.

4. The key to success is this: *don't let your child fall asleep in your arms*. Hold and comfort baby in your arms until she is drowsy and nodding off but not fully asleep. Since going to sleep is a learned phenomenon, you want her to learn how to go to sleep on her own. Parents who make the mistake of holding their children in their arms until they are dead weight and fully asleep inadvertently *weave themselves* into the tapestry of their children's sleep cycle. You and your body become part of the equation for your baby to get to sleep, and thus, when it's bedtime, *your baby will always need you to be there*. As one mother put it, "I have become my child's human pacifier."

5. Babies need to go down in their own cribs. When your baby reaches the point that she is drowsy and near the point of falling asleep in your arms, this is the moment to put her in her crib. In other words, your little girl must be fully cognizant that she is being put in her own crib, not your bed. *Cognizant* is the operative word here. Your baby must understand what's happening when she's being put to bed.

6. Anticipate that they will cry. Early on, when you're first getting into the sleep-training groove, children will undoubtedly cry when they are placed alone in their cribs. This is the usual and expected pattern, so don't be surprised. And don't be surprised either

with the intensity of their crying. They will be loud and adamant. Children can't talk at five months of age, but the meaning of this cry is unmistakable: "Pick me up *now!*"

7. Don't be bullied by the holler. The intensity of her cry will be downright intimidating, but hold tight. Allow her to cry for three to five minutes. Count off the time together on the clock with your spouse. Her sobbing will not hurt her, her psyche, her lungs, or her vocal cords. It only hurts your heart.

8. You can pick up your baby. After three to five minutes of this cacophonous harangue, if your baby is still crying—and she probably will be—go back into the room, pick her up, and comfort her. This is where I disagree with many other sleep experts. After these kinds of intense crying events, I believe it's natural (and reasonable) for a mother to want to comfort her child. I see no harm in this, and I believe it imparts to your child an understanding that she is loved and that she has not been abandoned.

9. It's important to calm your baby down again. After your child has wound herself up to this degree, it will take several minutes for her to relax and quiet down again. This is to be expected, so do not lose heart. If she has soiled or wet her diaper during this time, change her. And if you feel she is hungry or needs comfort, feed her again a small amount of either breast milk or formula, but whatever you do, don't let her fall asleep in your arms.

10. Get ready to do this all over again. When the storm is over and she has calmed down and she is again nodding off, put her down as before—drowsy, but cognizant that she is being put in her crib.

11. Expect her to cry intensely again. Most children will again cry, equally loud and equally intimidating. Allow her to cry, by the clock, for another three to five minutes, and then, like before, go to her, pick her up, and comfort her.

12. My sleep scheme allows children to cry for three to five

minutes, three times in a row, with parents picking them up to comfort and calm them between each crying period. After three episodes of three to five minutes of crying, I stretch it out to seven to ten minutes per crying episode. I again recommend three of these episodes with parents calming and comforting between each episode. Finally, after three three-to-five-minute episodes and three seven-to-ten-minute episodes, I tell parents to then allow their children to cry for twelve-to-fifteen-minute episodes thereafter until your child falls asleep.

13. Eventually, your baby will relent. The fatigue that she felt when the whole process began, sometimes hours before, will overwhelm her, and she'll ultimately fall fast asleep.

14. Whew! Oh, what a night! Sleep training is unbelievably stressful for most parents. It takes verve and courage to do it and do it right, but the payoffs are grand. When your baby finally quiets, revel in the peace and rest up for the next inning, because step 2 is coming soon.

15. Training your baby to go to sleep on her own is rarely a one-off experience. Generally, it takes between three and five nights of training before your baby understands the concept of going to bed alone, but when it is over, you have purchased for yourselves a whole new life. Ask parents who have been through the process and they will tell you that it is worth the effort and the pain of these few nights of crying.

STEP 2: Getting your baby through the night without feeds

1. Step 1 of my plan must be firmly in place before proceeding to step 2. Your first task is to make sure that your baby has learned step 1 and he is going to bed in his own crib in another room without a fuss.

2. Step 2 of my scheme should begin around six months of age

and only *after* your child has started having solid food meals. Like all of us, babies get hungry, but after they have begun solids, their hunger during nighttime hours will diminish, and they can make it through the night without a feeding.

3. After your baby has successfully learned step 1—that is, he is going to sleep at bedtime with little or no fuss—you can now start to train his middle-of-the-night awakenings. Like my recommendations in step 1, give him three to five minutes of crying before you go into the bedroom to quiet him. As before, when you do pick him up, comfort him, but now, *don't feed him.*

4. Like before, when you comfort him, he'll stop crying. After he has calmed down in your arms, remember not to let him fall asleep. Like step 1, put him back into his crib *cognizant* that he is going down.

5. He will probably cry again. If he again begins to cry, allow him to cry for three to five minutes. As with step 1, I allow children to cry for three to five minutes three times in a row, then seven to ten minutes three times in a row, and finally, twelve to fifteen minutes thereafter through the night.

6. If you hold your ground, babies will ultimately fall back to sleep without food. Physiologically speaking, at this age (six to seven months) babies *don't need* to be fed in the middle of the night.

7. Like step 1, step 2 requires about three to five days before a child learns that he is not going to be fed in the middle of the night. When this happens, you will then be able to gleefully declare to your friends and family, "Our baby sleeps *through the night!*" This is one of the great accomplishments of parenthood!

I have seen hundreds of families utilize this simple two-step plan with excellent outcomes, but it requires determination and persistence on the part of parents to employ it successfully.

When I instruct parents on this sleep program, I tell them to have a conversation with their babies before they embark. First, smile at their beloved daughters and sons, and then look them in their cute little eyes, and tell them, "Okay, now that you are a big girl [or boy], we're going to teach you how to sleep through the night." And then add, "And if it takes the entire night, we're going to do just that!"

That said, parents must be willing to spend all night going through my scheme and letting their children cry. *This never happens*, but this is the resolve parents must have to get the job done when they choose to do it.

> **SURPRISE:** According to recent studies, babies who sleep in their own rooms *sleep better* than those who sleep in the same room with their parents. For this reason, I recommend that children sleep in the same room with their parents for the first six months of life. After this, they will sleep better on their own, so put them in an adjacent room.

Mommies Need Sleep During the Newborn Stage Too

Q: How can I still feel rested and get enough sleep while my baby is a newborn?
A: There are several things you can do to assure you are getting as much sleep as possible while your baby is a newborn and still waking frequently at night.

- Sleep when the baby sleeps, even if that means taking a daytime nap and you are not a napper! You are adjusting to a very different way of life—the new world of parenting. Don't let the chores get in the way of taking a nap or going to bed early. Go easy on yourself! The laundry can wait.

- Take turns with your partner. Some couples find that sharing the midnight feedings helps them get the rest they need. You can do this by alternating nights (one night on, one night off) with Dad giving formula, or if you are breastfeeding, pump enough for a bottle so Dad can feed the baby once a night. Don't wait too long between breastfeedings, however, or you may end up engorged with clogged milk ducts.
- Keep your baby close. The quicker you can get your feeding done, the quicker you can all go back to sleep. If your baby is right next to your bed in a bassinet, you can get your baby fed and back to sleep in the shortest amount of time possible.
- Get some exercise. It can be tough to get a workout in when you're busy doing diaper changes and feedings, but you will benefit more from the time you spend sleeping if you get some exercise. Even twenty minutes a day can help you sleep better and feel more energized in the morning.

Eat healthy, and snack often. Ditch the junk food—it won't make you feel better and might even make you feel worse! Keeping a healthy, clean diet will help you feel good. Try to steer clear of sugary processed foods, and make sure you are giving yourself lots of fruits and vegetables. Eat plenty of healthy fats and high-protein snacks throughout the day for sustained energy. This will also help your body supply all the breast milk your baby needs and more.

3. Starting Your Baby on Solids

Good nutrition is of paramount importance to the growing young child. When babies are very young, mealtimes are simple. Mom and baby snuggle up together and either breastfeed or bottle-feed. These are wonderful moments of closeness and bonding. Some babies take both breast and bottle (with either Mom's pumped milk or formula) easily, which allows daddies the opportunity to feed their babies as well. Vitamin D and iron supplementation is recommended for babies during this time.

The First Thousand Days

The American Academy of Pediatrics (AAP) in 2018 put out a policy statement saying that a mother's prenatal nutrition and a child's nutrition during the first thousand days of life are "critical factors in a child's neurodevelopment and lifelong mental health." What a child is fed (both in utero and after birth) during these critical early years has long-term effects as these children advance into adulthood. Diseases such as obesity, hypertension, and diabetes are "programmed by nutritional status during this [one thousand-day] period." The statement goes on to say that "the most active period of neurologic development occurs in the first 1,000 days of life," which is the period "beginning at conception and ending at the start of the third postnatal year."

During the first weeks after delivery, feeding schedules tend to be erratic, but by four to six months of age, most babies have settled into a well-defined feeding schedule, and this is the time when nutritionists and gastroenterologists recommend that children start eating solid foods.

SURPRISE: Get Ready to Laugh

Starting little babies on solid foods provides some of the cutest moments of their young lives. Watching them experience—*and really like (and sometimes* not *like)*—solids is very funny, and these little entertainers put on a terrific show. So get the camera ready!

Just like sleep training, there are several food-introduction methods that mothers and fathers can follow when they begin solids for their babies. Like my recommendations for sleep training, my method for starting children on solid foods is not radically different from what other pediatricians recommend. That said, I have instructed thousands of mothers along these lines, and most of the babies I care for whose mothers and fathers have followed this basic plan have done well.

But if you find my recommendations confusing or if you need more details, my ultimate recommendation is *call your mother and ask her what to do!*

> **SURPRISE:** Children who share meals with their parents have fewer emotional problems when they are older and, as unrelated as it may sound, they actually perform better academically when they are older too.
>
> So eating with your children is one of my rules for parenting. Begin this habit when your children first begin solids, and follow this pattern throughout life.

Dr. Bob's Baby Feeding Plan

Here's what I tell parents when it comes time to start solids: I first want to know if their daughter is developmentally ready for feeding. The answers parents give to these four questions determine if their baby girl is ready to eat solid foods.

1. Is your daughter holding her head up well?
2. Does she open her mouth when food comes her way?
3. Has she been watching you eat with great interest?
4. Is she reaching out for your food?

If the answers to these questions are a clear *yes*, your baby is developmentally ready for food.

1. Begin feeding solids between four and six months. For children who are doing well on either breastfeeding or formula feeding, which means they are following the growth curve appropriately and not awakening hungry during the night, six months is the perfect time to begin solid feeds. For well babies who are younger than six months and who have been sleeping through the night but regress and begin to again awaken at night with apparent hunger, these younger-than-six-month-old babies should also start solids.

Children *can* safely start solid foods as young as four months of age. In fact, when I first started practicing pediatrics, this was the usual time pediatricians recommended introducing solid foods. Now we are waiting longer, and the general consensus in the pediatric community is to wait until six months. This delay allows for more gut maturation—and on a practical level, it saves the parents lots of cleanup. Feeding children is a messy proposition!

The American Academy of Pediatrics also recommends that breastfeeding be the sole source of nutrition for your child until six months. After solids have been started, the AAP recommends that breastfeeding continue until twelve months of age.

2. Start with a grain. Oatmeal, barley, and quinoa are good first foods for babies. I know that there are others who prefer to begin their patients on other foods like avocados or steamed vegetables. I have no problem with these other first-food choices, but there is no evidence that starting a child on one food over another has any clear health benefit.

3. Choose two times during the day, usually in the morning and early evening, when you would normally give your child either a breast feed or a bottle feed, to begin solids. These are times when you know your child is hungry. But *before* you give your baby milk at these feeding times, offer her two tablespoons of the solid food (cereal, vegetable, or fruit) of your choice.

After she finishes eating this solid meal, immediately wash down this feeding with either a breast or formula feed, remembering that since she is going to be partially satiated by the food she has just taken, she will require less milk at this feed than she would normally consume. By the way, when you begin your child on solid foods, you are, by definition, beginning the weaning process.

First Feeds

When babies first begin to eat, they may not get too much down. A strong *protrusion reflex* is present in every child, and they will frequently appear to be pushing out their food with their tongues. This diminishes with time as children learn to swallow textured foods, but with the first few feedings, don't expect them to take much. A teaspoon may be sufficient quantity for a novice feeder.

4. Follow a schedule of two solid feedings for one to two weeks. This allows the child to understand food textures and to learn the process of forming food boluses and swallowing solid foods.

5. Then, after one to two weeks, add a third solid food meal, usually at midday and again at a time when you would normally give your baby a milk meal. Instead of giving a cereal, I recommend that you try puréed vegetables like carrots, squash, or sweet potatoes.

6. Introduce one new food at a time. After you are up to three small feedings per day, I then recommend that moms and dads start introducing one new food, like a vegetable or a fruit, into their babies' diets every two or three days. The idea of individual introduction is to assess whether a child has an allergy to a particular food.

7. You can try white meats, like chicken, turkey, and fish, after your child has worked her way through several kinds of cereals, vegetables, and fruits.

The LEAP Study

Peanut allergy has recently doubled, increasing in the Western world among young children from 1.4 percent to 3 percent. A recent study from the United Kingdom called the LEAP Study (Learning Early About Peanut Allergy) that was recently published in the *New England Journal of Medicine* elucidated new evidence showing that babies who are introduced early to peanuts (around seven months of age) had significantly *fewer* allergies to peanuts at age five than those children who avoided peanuts early on. This study indicates that earlier exposure to "high-risk" foods diminishes allergy potential.

8. By nine months of age, your child should be on three meals a day. You also have plenty of liberty in what you can give to your baby. Introducing the whole egg, along with partially digested dairy products, like yogurt, kefir, and soft cheeses, is likewise okay. I also introduce ground red meat at this time.

Finally, at nine months of age, I also recommend introducing finger foods like small pieces of banana, Cheerios, scrambled eggs, well-cooked pasta, chicken that is finely diced and well cooked, and cut-up squash, peas, and potatoes.

9. At one year of age, parents can widen the array of foods and include whole, regular milk and honey in your babies' diets. By this time, your child should be at your table having the same foods that you have.

Food Allergies

The top eight foods that cause allergies in young children are:

- Dairy/milk
- Eggs
- Wheat/gluten
- Soy
- Peanuts
- Tree nuts (walnuts, cashews, almonds, etc.)
- Fish
- Shellfish

If you suspect food allergy (usually due to an immune reaction to a food protein) or food intolerance (a nonimmune reaction to a food, like lactose intolerance) with your baby, talk with your pediatrician.

There is good news coming on the allergy front. As a result of the LEAP study, and other studies that confirmed its findings, there are new products on the market that are designed to be introduced to your less-than-six-month-old child that will reduce childhood allergies to peanuts, milk, and eggs by up to 80 percent.

My observation over many years has been that for the first year, children are great eaters. They are eager for food at six months and accept most foods happily and graciously.

Unfortunately, as many mothers will tell you, during the second year of life, children frequently change. Their range of chosen foods narrows, and they develop clear aversions to many foods, but for now, enjoy their avid food interest.

Preventing Picky Eaters

If you avoid introducing processed foods into the diet from the start, your child will learn to enjoy eating a wide variety of fresh fruits, vegetables, and whole grains. This means *you* must also keep your diet free of junk food as well (at least while your baby is around!). If you are eating potato chips and ice cream, your baby is going to want some too. If you occasionally choose to indulge yourself, save it for when your baby isn't watching. For the most part, however, my recommendation is to keep *both* of your diets clean—if nothing else, for the sake of avoiding all the mealtime battles that will inevitably come your way later!

It's easy to fall into the trap of giving our kids convenience foods because they cut short the bother of preparing wholesome, homemade snacks. Handing your baby a bag of crackers is certainly easier than peeling a clementine or slicing some apples. Teaching your children to eat right takes a bit of work, but it's worth it in the long run. Your hard work will reward both you and your child for many years to come.

A Mommy Who Knows How to Get Her Girls to Eat Right

I recently had a mother and her three daughters in the office for their annual checkups. As I do with all my patients, I asked this mother if any of her children had food issues. She gave me a curious look and asked, "What do you mean?" I explained that many parents deal with food issues with their children and this was just one of the things I like to know about.

Her response took me off guard. "Dr. Hamilton," she said, "my children eat well because they have no choice in the matter. If they don't eat what I put in front of them, they go hungry." Needless to say, I was totally impressed with this mother's clear resolve. There was no rancor in her voice. She simply shared with me, in a quiet and matter-of-fact manner, her family's rules. And for the record, this woman is raising three lovely daughters who are healthy, eat a nutritious and balanced diet, and are delightful in every way.

Getting Patterns Established Pays Dividends Later

So to review, the three milestones that parents must work through during the first year are:

- Early scheduling
- Sleeping through the night
- The commencement of feeding

All three of these developmental landmarks come naturally and in their own time, but consistency, diligence to the task, and guidance speed the process and are required to establish healthy rhythms.

Successfully accomplishing these tasks when your child is young puts your sons and daughters on the right track as they grow and mature into the second year of life. Like adults, babies become creatures of habit very quickly. Guiding them into healthy life patterns now, when they are babies, will save you the time and effort (and headache) it takes to change and break bad patterns later.

The longer any one behavior is maintained (like awakening at three o'clock in the morning to feed), the more difficult it becomes to change it later. This is simply the nature of humans.

Having said that, when children are young, they are malleable; they're not old dogs who cannot learn new tricks—but children who have not been shaped at all in the first year are going to be a challenge.

And never forget where you are going after your baby's first birthday: you're heading smack-dab into the second year of life, which is capped off by the "terrible twos."

But that's a story for another day . . .

9

. . . . .

Embrace the Mundane—Have Fun with Your Baby and Enliven Your Child's Senses All at the Same Time!

The ancient Hebrews got it right. They understood the value of everyday experiences and mundane moments and the importance of making every minute count.

In Deuteronomy, the fifth book of the Torah, Moses urged the people of Israel to remember the words of the Lord. To aid them in the task, he commanded them to "tie" God's word as symbols on their hands, and to "bind them" to their foreheads. These outward signs of faithfulness helped the Hebrews to "fix" God's word, more importantly, on their hearts and minds.

Understanding that one faithful generation isn't enough, Moses, who clearly had his mind set on an unending legacy of faithful men and women, issued yet another command. He advised his people to teach God's words to their children. He then set the context in which this teaching was meant to occur. It wasn't a classroom with a chalkboard. Hebrew mommies and daddies were told to teach their children "when you sit at home and when you walk along the road, when you lie down and when you get up."

Essentially, what Moses was telling his people was this: every second of your life with your children can be a teaching moment.

Every moment of life counts. Those everyday times of life—the ones when you are sitting around your home or walking down the street, those chaotic moments before you get your kids to bed, and those brief, soft, and tender twinkles when they awaken in the morning—all these times with your children look like and may seem to be ordinary, but they are not. Instead, they're *extraordinary, precious, and highly consequential moments.* They turn out to be the *very* snippets of time we must use to teach our children how to live—which was understood, in ancient times, to be the responsibility of the parents.

SURPRISE: Your Child Will Think the Mundane Is Cool!

You may think your daily chores and mundane parts of life are nothing special, but your child will be filled with delight unloading the dryer or going grocery shopping with you. Not only will she love to be with you, her eyes will see the daily chores of life as fascinating and new.

New Eyes

By necessity, I recently had to walk (rather than drive) from my home to our local downtown area. It's only a 1.5-mile distance, but because I hadn't planned the time to walk into my morning schedule, I found myself mildly annoyed at having to take twenty-five minutes to make the otherwise rapid trip.

Within a block after stomping out the door, I realized that my immature and frosty attitude wasn't going to change the reality of my situation in the least, so I repented and decided to stop being a sixty-year-old brat and instead chose to play a mental game with myself. Rather than plodding down the street with my eyes fixed straight ahead, a bored victim of circumstances and blind to the wonder that surrounded me, I mindfully lifted my head, looked around, and sought to find something novel and lovely in every home and garden that I passed. I even stopped and smelled a couple of roses along the way.

As one may suspect, my attitude improved, and with this new perspective, another amazing thing happened. I found myself surrounded by beauty—from the pink-and-purple brocades of bougainvillea that cascaded over the walls of several yards to the black-eyed Susans that reflected the morning sun to the stout sycamores soaring high into the blue sky. The black-and-white neighborhood that I had driven through countless times and that I was planning on sullenly trudging through came alive with color.

Even the eclectic architecture caused my mind to wander afar. One English country manor–style house reminded me of the cobbled streets of Cambridge, England. A Spanish-style home stirred memories of a Guatemalan coffee *finca* I once visited. Finally, a modern, gray, and sharp-angled house planted me firmly on the face of the moon.

And then it was over. My mile-and-a-half trek—a course that I had driven many, many times before—zipped by painlessly. And it all happened because I opened my eyes and decided to look at things differently.

> *The ineffable inhabits the magnificent and the common, the grandiose and the tiny facts of reality alike. Some people sense this quality at distant intervals in extraordinary events; others sense it in the ordinary events, in every fold, in every nook, day after day, hour after hour. To them things are bereft of triteness.*
>
> —ABRAHAM JOSHUA HESCHEL, *THE WISDOM OF HESCHEL*

The Fresh Eyes of Children

To a baby, everything is fresh and new! The tasks that are normal to you, the humdrum things that you do every day, are *exciting* to your baby. As we all know, the chores of life are never ending, but tending to those duties with children at your side provides joyous opportunities to teach your young ones many things: the colors of the socks in the dryer, the names of vegetables at the store, what grass feels like after it has been mowed, and the names of the streets you pass on the way to the store.

As you engage your baby with these heretofore monotonous chores, the otherwise everyday moments of your day will be resurrected to you as well. Like the joy one feels when giving a tour of one's hometown to a visiting friend, so is the joy of seeing the mundane through the eyes of a child. You will see that your little someone is watching you—and he's taking notes too!

The simple errands and chores of life that we can find tiresome—picking up the dry cleaning, taking out the garbage, loading the dishwasher, or even shaving—these are the events that your children will find fascinating. And with every new thing that they see, they are growing and learning.

Consider this example: Think of the amazing sensory input that occurs when you bring your baby to the grocery store. This everyday errand affords your baby an unparalleled panoply of sensory input. They feel vestibular movement as you whisk and wheel them through the aisles in a grocery cart. They see the colorful cornucopia of products on the shelves and smell fresh fruits and vegetables along the way. They sense the coolness in front of the dairy shelves and ice cream freezers, feel the texture of a fresh peach, and finally, they'll hear whizzing cash registers as you check out.

And this doesn't include the oohs and aahs of the many who come up to adore your baby (and, of course, offer some vital advice on how they think you should raise her). All these seemingly simple things are feeding your child's brain and stimulating her cortex.

Eight Fun but Mundane Things to Do with Your Child

1. Play "this little piggy" as you get baby dressed in the morning or at diaper changes; use this perennial game to count baby's toes or fingers.
2. Blow bubbles in the bath, whip up a batch of bubbles with a little extra soap; be sure to blow them around baby, not near her face.
3. Make an obstacle course before you sit down on the couch to fold all those loads of laundry; put cushions, cardboard boxes, and pillows on the floor and show your crawling baby how to navigate over, under, and around them.
4. Follow the leader. As you sweep or vacuum the house, encourage baby to follow you, varying your speed; let baby catch you from time to time.
5. Count everything: steps on the way to the garage, windows in the hallway, toes going into shoes, apples into the shopping cart.
6. When bathing your baby, use plastic cups and bowls in the bath to pour, shake, dip, and swish.
7. Baby in a box: All those big Amazon boxes that arrive at your home every day can become toys. Put your baby in a cardboard box and push or drag him around the house.
8. Opposites: As you tidy a room, describe what you are doing. Turn a light switch off and on, off and on; put away a big toy and then a small one; put a toy above a table and then under it. Repetition is the key here.

Fill Your Home with Music

The universal, and what some consider as *mundane*, language of music has ancient roots in human societies and brings and binds people together like nothing else. Although music surrounds us in the modern world, music can also inspire our dreams, calm our fears, induce tears, elevate our spirits with unspeakable joy, and even pull us—sometimes against our own will—onto the dance floor. Singer Billy Joel once said that music is "an explosive expression of humanity." He's right! It's woven into our human DNA and is an ingredient to all the significant events of our lives. Just imagine a wedding without a processional, a graduation without a recessional, or a football game without the national anthem. Music adds to the fun, the excitement, the drama, and the elegance of every event.

So don't let your baby miss out. Let music be a vibrant part of your child's life from her first breath. Turn on your CD and turn up the volume. Even those rusty piano skills, a talent that might have lain dormant since high school, can be dusted off and reborn for the sake of your baby. Put all those tedious (and sometimes lonely) hours of practice to use entertaining your newborn.

This is because babies love *all* music, but they're particularly fascinated with *live* music, especially when it's played close at hand by someone they know. Watching the flying fingers of a musician and hearing a melody (and maybe a few groans, and plunks) from a live instrument enthralls and excites a child. You'll get some of your best-ever "gummy bear" smiles from your daughter when you play for her.

You can also bring your children to live music events, like church services or concerts at the park. Maybe your son won't make it through an entire Mahler symphony, but listening to and being among a congregation singing hymns will enrich him, and, for certain, he'll do just fine shimmying and shaking at the country fair hoedown.

The Devolved Concertmaster

When I was a teenager, I enjoyed playing the violin and as a senior in high school became the concertmaster of our local school symphony. It was a wonderful experience, but with the rigors of my college premedical studies and my subsequent medical school training, my violin virtuosity unfortunately peaked in the twelfth grade.

Though I don't play in any formal ensembles now, over the years I have enjoyed picking up my instrument and playing, though my playing doesn't always entertain others all the time. The unrefined squeaks that emanate from my fiddle have sometimes resulted in dogs howling and doors quietly being shut. But now, finally, I have found an audience that appreciates me and my violin playing: my grandchildren! *They love it when I play my violin!*

And so I do—and though nothing lasts forever, I can transfix them for twenty to thirty minutes at a stretch.

Amazingly, now my wife and even my children, who are some of the fiercest musical critics on the planet, *actually ask me to play!* Ah, 'tis so sweet to hear this request!

So I have reengaged with my fiddle for the sake of my grandchildren, and there is nothing more fun than playing for them.

Tips for Finding Baby-Friendly Live Music

- **Consider the venue:** Outdoor venues often have lots of space for you to stand near the back and walk around with your little one in a carrier. If you are going to an indoor event, sit near the back so you can exit quickly if your baby decides before you do that it's time to leave.
- **Consider the audience:** What type of audience will this performance draw? Will it be a family-friendly, smoke-free crowd?

: **Use ear protection when necessary:** Some live shows are meant to be louder than others, but just because a show is loud does not mean you can't bring your baby along for the ride. However, make sure you bring ear protection for your little one, preferably noise-canceling earmuffs, so you can assure no damage will be done to their hearing.

Sing to Your Baby

As much as young babies love instrumental music, babies particularly love singing, and they don't care if you sing in tune. I believe that the human voice is the most wonderful musical instrument in the universe, and all infants whom I've met agree. Little babies perk up and smile when their mommies start singing.

Research shows this to be true. According to a 2015 Canadian study cowritten by Sandra Trehub, Ph.D., "Singing is more effective than speech at keeping infants calm and delaying the onset of crying."

Newborns love a soothing lullaby, while older babies and preschoolers enjoy lively nursery rhymes or even your favorite songs on the radio.

Music Is Meant to Be Enjoyed Together

Another of the delightful aspects of music, and the reason parents should engage their child in music from the very start, is parents and children can enjoy music *together*. Unlike language, which is by its nature a to-and-fro interaction, music—including singing, playing it, or dancing to it—is done in synchrony with other people and is simultaneously appreciated by all who are listening and engaged.

The contemporaneous pleasure that music affords groups of people also has a deeper effect. It helps to build community. Enjoying music together bonds us one to another. As we enjoy a beat and sing together, there is a sense of commonality and connection that is unique. Studies show that the brain circuits responsible for controlling one's own actions are also involved in perceiving the actions of others. Those same "mirror neurons" that cause young infants to want to mimic their caregivers are also at work when it comes to music, compelling babies to join in with the beat.

Studies further show that performing actions like singing and dancing simultaneously with another person leads to a blurring effect between self and others *in the mind*. In other words, your brain begins to consider you and the others you are having fun with to be united into a communal larger self, which effectively promotes a sense of connection, both emotionally and psychologically. This self-blurring is particularly strong when people engage in repeated rhythmic movement like swaying to a beat. Rhythmic movements also release endorphins in the brain, which add to the pleasure of the moment and an enhanced emotional state.

So expose your babies to music. They'll love it, and you'll see them, even from an early age, rock to the beat. By the way, don't limit your baby to only one genre of music. Expose your child to all kinds of music, including classical, pop, and yes, *even country!* In doing so, you are opening their little minds and stimulating their brains.

Take Your Babies on a Visual Journey

But don't limit the awakening of your baby's senses with music; open their eyes too. Leonardo da Vinci believed that sight was the supreme sense and once wrote, "The eye, which is said to be the window of the soul, is the principal means by which the brain's sensory receptor may fully and magnificently contemplate the infinite works of nature." Da Vinci got it right. He was famous for extended periods of observing nature, such as the flight of birds and the patterns that currents of water produced.

From the first moments of life, your baby will be using her eyes to look around and understand the new world that she has been thrust into. As parents, our job is to keep that adventure alive with scenes of loveliness and novelty.

Show her pictures on walls—any walls, but especially the walls of your home. To this day, I vividly remember pictures and montages that hung in my childhood home when I was young. It doesn't really matter whether you have fine art or family snapshots, original oil paintings or bargain-store posters. The point is this: *Put something on your walls that will stimulate your child.*

And don't limit your baby's visual enlightenment to your home. Art museums allow babies in their doors too. No, your child won't understand the differences between the artistic styles of Rembrandt versus Van Gogh, but she will appreciate the colors and the images as much as anyone of any age.

Photo albums or pictures of family members are also wonderful tools to capture the imagination and visually stimulate young children. Make a photo album showing members of your family and close friends to share with them. If you have craft skills, make a simple mobile for the kitchen displaying family images. Your baby will love it.

It Seems Mundane, but Talking to Your Baby (a Lot) Is Important

Talking is about as mundane as you can get, but your words will stimulate your baby's brain. Just talking—or as one pediatrician I know put it, "narrating your life and actions"—will have a direct influence on your child's understanding of the world and even enhance her IQ.

Studies show that babies who hear more words in the formative months and years of their lives perform better on intelligence tests. This is because parents who talk a lot to their children expose them, over time, to literally *millions* of more words than laconic parents. Babies store this oral input into the temporal cortex of their brains. A baby who hears millions of words spoken to him personally has an expanded and richer trove of verbal experiences and thus becomes more adept verbally than a child who lacks this kind of input. In baseball terms, babies who are raised in loquacious households live life in a verbal batting cage. They are fortunate to hear and digitally digest hundreds of *more* hours of verbal data than babies who don't experience this kind of intense aural input.

It therefore follows that talking to babies early on carries with it the benefit of them learning to speak and develop their language skills earlier. Author Jill Stamm put it like this: "Feeding your baby with words is as essential as nourishing them with food." So talk to your baby as much as you can: narrate your activities, explain what you are doing, read books, converse in front of him— we aren't after understanding, just exposure to language.

Speaking in Tongues

As a mom or dad, you are about to begin speaking a new language. It's the language of your infant. As you *goo* and *gaa* with your wee one, you will find yourself lapsing into odd linguistic behaviors. You may even find yourself speaking in tongues! These utterances may even surprise you, but they are normal.

The language of parents speaking to babies is called *parentese*. It is an animated, high-pitched, drawn-out, and clearly enunciated "slanguage" that we find ourselves speaking to our babies. By slowly articulating each word, we teach our children to hear the individual sounds, called *phonemes*, that make up each word. Phonemes are the building blocks of oral language, and later, they form the basis for deciphering the written word as well.

Here is how parentese works: Vowels are prolonged, and there's energy and excitement in every word spoken. Rather than saying in your usual voice, "Oh, sweetie, look at the ball," you will find yourself gushing, "*Oooh, sweeetieee, loooook at the baaaall!*" Parentese uses real words and real sentences and real ideas. It's simply a variation of the rhythm and the drawing out of sounds that makes it unique.

Studies show that parentese, which is a universal phenomenon, matches perfectly what young minds need to hear as they process language—in pitch, in cadence, and in clarity.

Parentese Isn't Baby Talk

Parentese is not baby talk! *Baby talk* is nonsensical babbling that mimics the early protolanguage of infants. This is certainly good and fine for parents to do, and it comes naturally . . . and it's silly and fun.

Parentese, on the other hand, is standard English (or the native language of the home), but it is spoken in a clear and animated fashion that breaks down each word into its individual parts.

Parentese aside, yours may be a home where many languages are spoken. It's a myth that children cannot learn second or even third languages simultaneously. They can do it very well. It is best for adults to use the language that they are the most fluent in speaking when conversing with their babies.

I have many families in my practice whose first language is not English. I encourage them to teach their native languages to their children, and most of my families wisely choose to do just that. Babies are capable of learning more than one language and even become highly competent in knowing to whom to speak which language. Multilingual homes enrich a child and help your child by helping to develop her communication skills.

Reading to Your Baby

Reading to babies is just as important as talking to babies, *even when they are newborns*. When you read to them, they are listening to the ebb and flow of your voice, and these spoken words are all being recorded in their little brains. The mellifluous sound of your voice also brings comfort and solace to your baby.

The American Academy of Pediatrics (AAP) recommends daily reading to your child beginning from birth. According to the academy, "Families should be strongly encouraged to sit down and read to their child to foster their child's cognitive and language development."

Reading to your babies from birth also allows for special moments to snuggle with your infant and plant positive emotional memories surrounding the spoken and written word. If you cultivate this pattern during the early months, as your child grows, she will independently seek out books on her own and, more often than not, become an avid reader herself, which is something all parents should encourage.

Reading with Your Baby: How to Help Her Learn

- Use small board books that your baby can easily hold.
- Talk about the pictures with your little one.
- Sing the text to keep your child's attention.
- Play peekaboo with lift-the-flap books.
- Help your baby touch and feel with texture books.
- Cuddle up and read with emotion.
- Ask your baby questions and then answer them for her.
- Plan a special reading time each day, even though it may last only for a couple of minutes. Let your child be the barometer of when to stop. As children mature, the length of time that they show interest will increase.

And don't forget to include poetry in your reading mix. Even very young children delight in the rhyme and rhythm of poetry. Sharing the spoken word in all its rich and wonderful forms lays the foundation for your baby's language development.

The Five Rs of Early Education

- *Reading* together as a daily, fun, and family activity.
- *Rhyming* together through playing, talking, singing, and cuddling often throughout the day.
- *Routines* for meals, play, and sleep, which help children know what to expect and what is expected of them.
- *Rewards* for everyday successes, understanding that praise from those closest to a child is a very potent reward.
- *Relationships* that are nurturing, reciprocal, purposeful, and lasting, which are the foundation of healthy early brain and child development.

Get Out of the House and into Nature

Another mundane thing you can do with your young baby is open the front door and take him for a walk! Allow your infant to feel the wind in his face, the chill of the morning, the warmth of the sun, the cold of snow, and the wetness of rain.

Bring him to the park to watch the ducks in the pond, see other children play, and hear fallen leaves rustle along the ground. Allow him to touch the earth. Take him to the beach and let him feel sand slip through his fingers and enjoy the pleasure of waves lapping at his feet. Bring him with you into a pool and let him feel that unique buoyancy that water provides. Take him to the zoo to watch the monkeys swing and hear the lions roar.

I tell my patients' parents that I think babies and young children should "live outdoors" as much as possible. I make this recommendation because there are few things that babies love more than to be outside. I even use "outdoor therapy" for tough cases of colic. For many of my fussy babies, there is nothing that calms them other than a walk through the neighborhood. But even non-colicky babies benefit and enjoy the excitement that comes by being outdoors.

Fewer Kids Are Enjoying the Outdoors in the Western World

Researchers who study child and family behavior patterns have recently reported some disturbing news. They've found that there is a growing trend for America's children to live and stay indoors more than ever before. The loss of outdoor activities represents the dark side of American prosperity as our gadgets and televisions seem to be separating us further and further from the earth.

As hard as it is to believe, a recent study by the National Wildlife

Federation shows that American children are now spending fewer than thirty minutes *per week* playing outside. Adults are no better, preferring the order of their inside, contained world to the randomness of nature.

This lack of outdoor activity is fostering what researchers call *biophobia*, which is defined as "fear of the natural world." Researchers are finding that both adults and their children are becoming fearful of the real world. For some children, hearing a flock of noisy birds or feeling a strong wind induces a surge of anxiety that triggers a fight-or-flight stress response. Make sure your baby doesn't suffer from biophobia! Take her outdoors and enjoy the wonder of the natural world.

Part of the retreat from nature is driven by fear of children getting exposed to viruses and bacteria. Microbiologists B. Brett Finlay and Marie-Claire Arrieta, authors of the book *Let Them Eat Dirt*, put it this way in a *Wall Street Journal* essay: "Never before have babies and children grown up so cleanly."

But there is a negative side to this obsession with cleanliness. Being scrubbed clean, inside and out, cuts back on what scientists called the *natural microbiota*, those good bacteria that help humans, from the very beginning of their lives, modulate their immune and metabolic systems. Our inside and outside microbiota protect us from a host of ills like asthma, allergies, and inflammatory bowel diseases. There is also a relationship between a healthy microbiota and metabolic diseases like obesity and diabetes.

Seeing this parental war against naturally occurring, harmless bacteria, Finlay and Arrieta concluded that parents who prevent their babies and children from following their "innate impulse to get dirty" are shielding them from "the microbial exposure that is essential for the development of a healthy immune system."

Susan Lynch, Ph.D., from University of California, San Francisco, affirms this data and advocates that even newborns need to "get dirty." Her studies show the microorganisms that infants encounter when they are squeezed through the vaginal tract benefit them. Dr. Lynch has found that vaginal birth, breastfeeding, and having an outdoor dog in the house all enhance the richness of the microbiota in the newborn gut. If the colonization of these bacteria is impeded, even during the early days of life, the chance of a child having allergies and asthma increases threefold. According to Dr. Lynch, analyzing the composition of the gut flora in the first months of life allows doctors to predict within a reasonable measure which children will have allergies at two years of age and asthma at four years of age.

Six Scientifically Proven Reasons Why Taking Kids Outdoors Is Good

1. Improves vision: Children who spent time outdoors have less myopia (an inability to see distant objects, which is referred to as *nearsightedness*). A study from the National Center for Children's Vision and Eye Health found that 4 percent of children ages six to seventy-two months have myopia.
2. Provides vitamin D: Natural sunlight provides vitamin D. (The vitamin D_3 hormone is synthesized in the skin from its precursor, 7-dehydroxycholesterol, when the skin is bathed in sunlight.) Vitamin D is important for bone formation and mineral homeostasis. Individuals who are vitamin D deficient develop rickets and bone thinning.
3. Promotes healthy sleep patterns: Children who spend time outdoors develop better sleep patterns than sedentary children.
4. Offers clean air: Fresh air is one of the benefits of outdoor life.
5. Gets kids standing and moving: Exercise expends energy and helps your child develop motor skills.
6. Decreases stress: Studies have shown that older children who spend more time outside experience less stress than children who do not.

Natural impulses seem to tell babies that getting yucky outside is good. Maybe this is the reason babies love the outdoors so much! Other than getting dirty, the vastness of the sky and the vibrancy and adventure of the outdoors challenges them. So get your babies outdoors and let them get dirty too. They'll love it, and in the end, they'll be healthier for it.

SURPRISE: Bad Weather Doesn't Have to Keep Your Baby Inside

There is an old Swedish saying: "There is no bad weather, only bad clothes." Rain, snow, and wind can deter even the hardy, but don't let gray skies subdue you and your baby.

I'm not recommending taking baby out during lightning storms, hurricanes, or tornadoes, but when one is dressed for the occasion, most weather—even the most inclement—can be fun! I still fondly remember the joy of stomping through mud puddles in rubber rain boots as a child.

Mundane Kids' Play Is a Learning Opportunity

It has been said that "play is children's work." Before leaving our list of seemingly mundane endeavors, it's worth spending a moment to discuss play. Children gain many benefits from play. When young children play with objects, they are required to think through and solve problems. Playtime enhances and optimizes a child's cognitive, physical, social, and emotional development and gives babies an opportunity to test their understanding about how the world works. Through games and puzzles, they increase their problem-solving skills and even their language skills.

When children play with different-shaped objects, for example, they gain a better understanding of shape, size, and texture. They also learn that they cannot put a square peg in a round hole!

Play also allows children to master skills that enhance self-confidence and the ability to recover from setbacks. You see it in the pride children sense when they build a tower of blocks and the disappointment they show when their tower tumbles to the ground.

> *Play connects children with their imagination, their environment, their parents and family and the world.*
> —JONA K. ANDERSON-MCNAMEE AND SANDRA J. BAILEY,
> "THE IMPORTANCE OF PLAY IN EARLY CHILDHOOD
> DEVELOPMENT"

Parental involvement in play, especially with infants, is likewise important. Playing with your baby enhances bonding, increases communication, allows for teachable moments, and provides a format to assist in problem solving.

When playing with your babies, there is no reason to puzzle about how or with what toys you need to have to play with your child, and there's no need to go to the toy store. Children love simple, everyday items that are found around your home. Anything that your child finds interesting is a toy.

The kitchen is a great place to start. Mixing spoons, pots, pans, and Tupperware bowls that nest together all provide great entertainment.

Babies also love mirrors, especially around three to four months of age. There is nothing more exciting to a young infant than the human face, even if it is her own. Prop an unbreakable mirror in her crib or nearby on a wall where she can see her own image. It will keep her more occupied while on her tummy, which babies generally do *not* like early on. While playing with her in front of a mirror, point to her features and touch her, saying something like, "Look at your nose!"

Gotcha Games

As early as six months of age, children understand the concept of object permanence and love to play "gotcha" games and peekaboo. Like everyone, children love surprises. Young children thrill in the anticipation of "gotcha" and take joy in being caught (and tickled). Look for ways to create happy surprises with your baby.

And while you are having a good time, don't forget to blow raspberries on your baby's tummy! This is one of the true joys of parenthood, and babies love it too. Young babies are not quite ready for real roughhousing, but a raspberry or two on baby's tummy is "proto-roughhousing." It's fun, and your baby will love it!

The Right to Play

Play has been recognized by the United Nations as a human right for every child.

States Parties recognize the right of the child to rest and leisure, to engage in play and recreational activities.
—UN CONVENTION ON THE RIGHT OF THE CHILD, 1989

Floor Time

Dads who play with their young children during the first year often find themselves spending time on the floor (on all fours), howling and barking like a dog. This is exactly what daddies are supposed to do. Your baby will love this more than you can possibly imagine, even though you will undoubtably annoy your partner and the neighbors. This is all part of the gentle rough-and-tumble, wild abandon that I thoroughly and heartily endorse. Remember too that baby girls and baby boys are well constructed. They bend before they break.

These are the moments when babies will feel *your* delight! They will sense that you *too* are having a grand time. From this, even though they will not remember the moment, an impression is being made: a warm and positive deposit has been made into their emotional bank accounts. These are the origins of positive and affirming emotional memories that are deeply imbedded in the hearts and souls of all humans.

The Different Types of Play

- Unoccupied Play: A child is not playing but observing.
- Solitary (Independent) Play: A child is playing alone.
- Onlooker Play: A child is observing other children who are playing.
- Parallel Play: Two or more children play next to each other without engaging each other.
- Associative Play: Two or more children play next to each other and engage each other through communication.
- Social (Cooperative) Play: When all the above types of play come together and two or more children play together and interact with each other.
- Motor/Physical Play: This includes any type of active play, like throwing a ball or riding a bike.
- Constructive Play: Any activity that teaches a child about manipulation, building, and fitting things together.
- Competitive Play: Play that involves rules and turn taking, like a simple board game or sport.
- Fantasy (Dramatic) Play: Imaginative play like "dress up," "doctor," or "restaurant," involving role-playing, cooperation, and language development.

Play allows for more creativity, imagination, dexterity, and socialization through work in groups, to share, negotiate, come to solutions, resolve conflicts, and to become self-advocates through self-reflection and decompression.

—*PEDIATRICS* MAGAZINE, JANUARY 2007 (VOL. 119, ISSUE 1)

Downtime and Boredom Are Okay

We live in a world of plugged-in people. Walk down the street, ride an elevator, or jump on the subway and look at the people around you. Everyone seems to have their earbuds in place, engaged in something. And it never ends. This endless electronic stimulation leaves little space for contemplation, reflection, and creativity—or boredom, for that matter. For babies, this is not good. It's healthy and critical for them to have *scheduled* unscheduled downtimes when they are allowed to play alone, without structure.

Charles Dickens, one of the greatest and most productive writers in the English language, had a habit of working from 9:00 A.M. till 2:00 P.M. and then venturing off on his own downtime, which took the form of long walks through the streets of London. He once wrote, "If I couldn't walk fast and far, I should just explode and perish." It was during these long walks that Dickens's creativity was ignited and his books were "written."

Giving babies this kind of quiet time to reflect and play alone, even though it may not appear to be productive, is extremely valuable. It allows them to ponder through and consolidate the activities of the day and allows them time to discover their environment without distraction.

Boredom is one of those human feelings that nobody particularly enjoys. It represents a dissatisfaction and, for some, a profound weariness with the present. But for most people, boredom creates in an intense sense of restlessness and angst.

So what happens when people and babies are bored? They cast about to escape their plight. When children feel bored, they become creative. They look around for something to capture their attention and their imagination. They find something to grab, a toy to play with, an image to study. In other words, boredom stimulates creative thinking and action. This happens in babies as much as it happens in adults. Writer Thomas Kersting, in his book *Disconnected*, wrote, "Boredom is to your brain what weight lifting is to your muscles." He calls boredom "mental fertilizer" and decries the urge of parents to fill every moment of a child's life, including young babies, with some sort of external stimulation, particularly electronic stimulation.

> *A hurried, overly pressured education that is focused on academic preparation and an overly scheduled lifestyle are interfering and interrupting the ability of children to have "child-driven" play.*
>
> —*PEDIATRICS* MAGAZINE, JANUARY 2007 (VOL. 119, ISSUE 1)

You Are Your Baby's Enrichment Program

Mommies and daddies who spend time with their children doing normal, everyday, mundane things *are* their children's enrichment program! Engaging and sharing with your children the routines of daily living and enlivening their five senses to the wonders that are in our world is all your children need during the first formative year of life.

So have fun and embrace the everyday moments of life. Take a lesson from Moses by teaching your child how to live "when you sit at home and when you walk along the road, when you lie down and when you get up." Here's how I paraphrase Moses's advice to the parents of my patients: "Put your kid in your back pocket and take them with you wherever you go!"

Instruct them about how life is *really lived* by including them in all the mundane events that each day brings, and as they watch you go about your daily tasks, take heart knowing that you are helping your baby learn and grow in the best possible way!

10

. . . . .

The Two-Parent Team

Secret #5: Moms and Dads Are *Equally* Important When Raising a Baby

Child rearing is an immersion in caring for the needs of another, very helpless individual. It's a time when men and women, by necessity, must dive into the task of caring for their *new* love. It's a time for selfless giving, and both moms and dads have unique roles to play in this great adventure of the first year of life with baby.

Mommies

Let's start with the mother. She has just gone through one of the most challenging and life-altering experiences that life delivers up. After a baby comes, a woman's goals, focus, emotions—even her body—will be different.

The changes in a new mother start in her brain, which undergoes actual physical alteration during gestation. As writer Adrienne LaFrance put it, "Pregnancy tinkers with the very structure of [a mom's] brain." Reconfigurations occur in the prefrontal cortex, midbrain, and parietal lobes. These changes can be seen when functional MRI studies are done. We have already learned that feeling "maternal" isn't an illusion. The emotional changes that a mother feels are a consequence of both *hormonal* and *brain* architectural alterations that take place during pregnancy.

The amygdala is a structure in the brain that processes memory and originates emotions like anxiety, aggression, and fear. After delivery, the amygdala grows and increases its number of binding sites for oxytocin, the "love hormone," which surges during pregnancy. With this increase in size, the amygdala, under the influence of oxytocin, becomes the epicenter for maternal-infant bonding.

> Writing about oxytocin, Erica Komisar, the author of the book *Being There*, calls oxytocin the "trust" and "bonding" hormone. "The more a mother engages with her baby, the more oxytocin she produces; the more oxytocin she produces, the more she bonds with her child; in other words, the more you love your baby, the more you can love your baby."

The Changes in a Woman's Body After Delivery

As well as the brain, physiological changes before and after childbirth affect virtually every organ of a woman's body, from the heart to the kidneys to the skeletal system.

The first step toward postdelivery recovery is the uterus shrinking back to its pre-pregnancy size. As soon as the placenta is delivered during the "third stage" of labor, involution of the uterus begins. The postdelivery uterus is about the size of a softball and weighs two pounds. In a little over six weeks, it squeezes down to its pre-pregnancy weight of two to three ounces and tucks itself back into a woman's pelvis below the pubic bone.

Many women experience pain in the postdelivery period, espe-cially if an episiotomy (a surgical incision that more readily allows for the delivery of the baby's head) was done or if there was perineal tearing. The greater the injury that occurred, the more bruising, swelling, and tenderness is present. Walking, sitting, urinating, and defecating may be painful. Sexual activity is generally not rec-ommended before six weeks after delivery.

Breastfeeding!

During pregnancy, many changes are occurring in women's breasts that gear them up to provide the perfect food for their babies at the exact moment it is needed. Within the first two months of pregnancy, the newly pregnant mother's breasts begin to enlarge as blood flow increases and glandular tissues enlarge. A mother's nipples become tender and larger, and the areolae (the surround-ing pigmented area around the nipples) expand and darken. By the end of the first trimester, a mother's breasts are proliferating with new milk ducts and milk-producing glands, which replace the fatty and supportive tissue of the nonpregnant breast.

After delivery, estrogen and progesterone decline quickly, while prolactin, the hormone that stimulates breast milk pro-duction, increases. The more the infant suckles, the more milk is produced. A mother's milk production works along the simple principle of supply and demand. Milk supply increases as her baby's stomach volume increases.

Q: *What happens to prolactin levels when a mother is not breast-feeding?*
A: Non-breastfeeding mothers see their prolactin levels return to normal (non-lactating) levels within one to two weeks after delivery, and menstruation will resume seven to nine weeks after delivery.

Breastfeeding delays both ovulation and thus menstruation as well. If you breastfeed exclusively for the first six months of your baby's life, you are unlikely to ovulate or become pregnant—but caution is advised. It doesn't always work out that way!

Another significant change that happens in the body of a post-delivery mother is weight loss. There is an immediate weight loss of ten to thirteen pounds with the delivery of the baby, placenta, amniotic fluid, and blood loss. Shortly after birth, a natural diuresis (excess urine loss) results in another five to eight pounds of weight loss. Finally, another two to three pounds are shed within a few weeks due to the uterus shrinking. Younger mothers with lower pre-pregnancy weights lose weight quicker than older moms. Adipose (fat-storing) tissue gained during pregnancy is lost more slowly, usually over a period of three to six months.

Mom's First Task: Recovery

In the first days and weeks after delivering a baby, a mother's hair may be thinner due to hormone changes; she might be sweating more as the body deals with excess fluid; her uterus has not shrunk yet, and a baby bump will still be visible. Her body has changed, and it will take some time for her pre-pregnancy body to return.

So one of the very first responsibilities a mother must accomplish after the birth of her child is *recovery*. Yes, it's also a mother's job to nourish and care for her baby, but if she pushes herself too hard too fast, it makes recovery from birth longer and more difficult.

The physical and mental changes that a new mommy experiences make for a wild ride. They are difficult to negotiate and contend with for any new mom, but this is where new dads come in!

Daddies

While all this is happening with Mom, Dad may be watching and wondering where he fits in. For some men, the process of pregnancy, childbirth, and breastfeeding is a fully feminine and foreign phenomenon. Many men engage the process with mixed emotions. They see that their partners—and with this, their lives together as a couple—are changing quickly.

"Baby making" happens when men and women find each other and fall in love, but actually *making a baby* is a task for a woman's body. For the guys watching their partners going through the process, it's like seeing the aurora borealis, a harvest moon, and a total eclipse of the sun all rolled into one human, double-rainbow experience. So, while moms are going through the nine months of this star-spangled, gestational extravaganza, dads are charged with the much less dramatic role of being supportive.

Dad's Hormones Are Raging Too!

But there's a lot more to it than men know. There are also *unseen hormonal changes* happening in men that most guys (and gals) are completely unaware of. Like the hormonal changes that happen in women, men—at least those men who live together with their partners during gestation—undergo an internal hormonal storm that is preparing them for their future role of being daddies. Referred to in the neurobiology field as *biobehavioral synchrony*, the contemporaneous hormonal changes that occur in *both* men and women during gestation represent a stealth mother-father codependency that is important for child rearing in biparental, monogamous animal species.

Things hormonally begin changing for men around the end of the first trimester into their partners' pregnancies. God, in his infinite wisdom, surreptitiously built into pregnancy an arrangement between men and women, ultimately for the health and well-being of the newborn on the way. In biblical terms, "the two shall become one flesh." In medical terms, men begin to hormonally look a little more like women.

The hormonal changes that men experience start with the ultimate male hormone: *testosterone*. Known as the "macho" hormone, testosterone is associated with sexual partner seeking and aggressive conduct in men. These classical male behaviors are not necessarily conducive for good fathering, and thus, unbeknownst to most to-be daddies, testosterone levels begin to tumble during pregnancy, especially during the final trimester. They continue to be low for several months after delivery. Researchers studying this phenomenon suggest that this reduction in testosterone results in less risk-taking (a daddy is going to be needed by both Mommy and the baby, so this is not a great time for Dad to die) *and* an increase in what most would consider more "feminine" behavior—namely, *nurturing*. Men are clearly capable of nurturing, but they do a better job of it when they are not under the influence and taunted by elevated testosterone levels. So nature solved the puzzle and helped men out by slowing down the factory.

Another hormone, one that we are well acquainted with as affecting mothers, also shows up to change the nature of men too. The famous "love" hormone, oxytocin, that so positively influences nursing mothers to bond with their babies also increases in the serum of fathers, and, as it does in women, oxytocin prods men to bond with their babies. For men, the oxytocin increase is minuscule compared to that of a nursing mother, but even a slight boost in oxytocin levels in men intensifies their sense of devotion toward their baby. Oxytocin increases as a graded response; the more involvement a dad has with his child, the higher oxytocin rises. As one might expect, dads who spend minimal time with their newborn children don't get this oxytocin bump and sadly will therefore not have the same intensity of closeness with their newborns. For dads, inducing an oxytocin bump should be worth fighting for! (Stephanie Pappas, "The Science of Fatherhood: Why Dads Matter," NBC News, June 19, 2012.)

Another hormone, prolactin, known to induce milk production in women, also increases in men. Made in the brain, this hormone in men causes them to become more alert and responsive to the cries of their babies.

Finally, still yet another hormone is active in the postpartum daddy. Vasopressin, sometimes known as the "monogamy" hormone, causes men to bond more fervently with their *partners*, become more jealous for the mother of their child, and thus more apt to guard and defend both mom and baby in the case of emergency.

Couvade Syndrome

Scientists have described a rare but unique constellation of symptoms that occur in some men who are cohabitating with a pregnant woman. Called *Couvade syndrome* or *sympathetic pregnancy*, it is regarded by most doctors as psychosomatic. Men with this syndrome mirror their partners' pregnancies with weight gain, morning sickness, and disturbed sleep patterns during pregnancy.

What's a Dad to Do?

Since breastfeeding occupies a big portion of caring for a newborn, biology dictates that mothers end up doing the bulk of the work with their babies early on. However, there's still plenty for dads to do to help care for babies, though some men feel ill at ease with the supporting role into which they've been cast. As one comedian quipped to his wife when she asked him to watch their newborn baby, "Just because you gave birth to a baby hardly qualifies *me* to start caring for one!"

But dads *do* have work to do. It's different work because moms and dads are uniquely different. As one writer put it: "Gender equal, but gender different." This becomes abundantly clear to any couple who has ever parented a child together.

But for those who ask, "Am I up for the job?" I assure them that they are and there are plenty of important reasons for dads to *want* to play their part.

Researchers who study families show clearly something that we all know intuitively—namely, dads who are intimately involved with their children have a huge influence on their children through-out life. Ronald Rohner, director of the Center for the Study of Interpersonal Acceptance and Rejection at the University of Con-necticut, says, "Knowing that kids feel loved by their father is a better predictor of young adults' sense of well-being, of happiness, of life satisfaction than knowing about the extent to which they feel loved by their mothers."

Dads' involvement in the lives of their children also increases their overall "stick-with-it-ness", a trait that Brigham Young Univer-sity researchers called *persistence*. Fathers' involvement with their children increased this quality in their children.

So here are a couple of ways dads can make a difference the first year of life with their babies:

- **Encouragement:** The first thing you can do for your partner is applaud! Tell her how proud you are of her and how honored you are to have a partner like her. Tell her how beautiful she is. Encourage her to breastfeed, and make yourself available to do whatever needs to be done—from getting a glass of water to making a meal. Studies show that dads who encourage their partners to breastfeed see exactly that. Their partners breastfeed their babies at higher rates than moms who don't receive support and encouragement from their partners—and this makes for happier and healthier babies!

- **Spend Time with Your Baby:** Do your half of the parenting workload by spending time with baby. Pick up your baby, hold him skin-to-skin, and enjoy *lots* of time with him. Look him in the eyes and tell him that you love him, but remember too that his focal length is short, so stay close to his face.

- **Baby Dates:** Dates don't have to be reserved only for your significant other. You can also "date your baby." Plan to spend one-on-one time with your little one as much as possible. This could be a daily walk around the block, a trip to the park, or simply a special time to cuddle. These "baby dates" give your partner some precious moments to rest and will further bond you with your newborn.

- **Diaper Changes:** Studies of postdelivery couples show that dads who share the dirty duty of diapers enhance their marriage in the long term. Not only will changing your baby's soiled diapers help take some of the pressure off Mom, it gives Dad more time to connect with baby through caring for him or her. One mother I know told me that she never touched a dirty diaper until her daughter was walking! Here's how she put it: "I was at the beck and call for breastfeeding. He was at the beck and call of what came out the other end!"

- **Feedings:** If possible, help your partner with feeding the baby by using pumped breast milk in a bottle or formula if she has chosen to supplement. Share the burden of night-time feedings this way; parenting is a twenty-four-hour-per-day job for everyone.

- **Baby Massages:** Give your baby a gentle massage! When you do, not only does he feel loved, studies show that massages benefit his sleeping and digestion as well.

- **Household Chores and Meals:** While this one is perhaps a rather obvious suggestion, it's important to take seriously. Prepare a meal for Mommy, do the dishes, and fold the laundry, even if these aren't usually on your to-do list. It's all hands on deck. While you may not be directly interacting with your baby through these chores, you are making sure the household runs, and that is good for *everyone*.

The Dreaded Baby Blues and More

In addition to helping to care for the new babe, dads also need to take special care of their partners during the newborn stage. Along with the biological fireworks that women experience, the period immediately after delivery can be an emotionally volatile time for many new moms. Nearly 70 percent of postpartum mothers go through a period of emotional letdown, otherwise known as the "baby blues," and up to 13 percent of recently delivered moms have significant depression. Fortunately, for most moms, postpartum blues passes within two weeks.

During these days, however, dads must be the emotional rock their partners need if they are being hammered by whacked-out hormone surges. I have many amazing women in my practice who shoulder great responsibility and are highly accomplished yet find themselves overwrought with emotion and brimming with tears in the postpartum days. This is not a rarity.

I think most postpartum mothers recognize how painfully vulnerable they are. The days after delivery are some of the most exposed and raw moments in the life of a woman. How their partners react during this time is important. Even though a postpartum mother may not act quite like herself, she nevertheless will remember every word spoken to her. For many men, this is a baptism by fire into the art of nurturing, and many times, the best thing a guy can do is exude kindness, maintain a calm spirit, and, to employ a biblical injunction, "be quick to listen and slow to speak." For the great majority of mothers, the situation is temporary, but how dads support and help their partners during this period is important both in the short term and in the long term as well.

Postpartum Depression

Postpartum blues are different from postpartum depression. Up to 70 percent of new moms suffer from the "baby blues." This emotional state peaks between two and five days after delivery and shows itself in excessive weepiness, sadness, mood lability, irritability, and anxiety. Symptoms do not seriously impair the ability of the mother to care for her newborn and generally resolve spontaneously by two weeks.

Postpartum depression, on the other hand, is more recalcitrant and includes symptoms such as pervasive depressed mood, diminished interest or pleasure in all or most activities, either significant weight loss or weight gain, insomnia or excessive sleeping, fatigue, feelings of worthlessness, excessive guilt, and suicidal ideation. Postpartum depression is estimated to affect 6–13 percent of women. Sleeplessness in the postpartum period plays a significant role in the cause of this phenomenon.

Postpartum depression is a serious medical issue and should be reported to a mother's obstetrician during postpartum follow-up appointments.

One Postpartum Mother with the Baby Blues

One mom in my practice, a successful lawyer, was hit particularly hard by the postpartum emotional roller coaster. Every morning when I saw her on my rounds, no matter what I said to her about her baby, she would burst into uncontrolled sobbing. When I told her she had a lovely baby, she sobbed. When I explained why her baby had a rash, she wept. When I shared with her that I thought her baby looked like the daddy, she welled with tears.

Since she had had a cesarean section delivery and thus was in the hospital for a longer period, this weeping scenario went on for several days. Finally, on the day she was scheduled to go home, I came into her room and said with a broad smile, "*Don't cry!*" She laughed momentarily, understanding the humor of my "command," but then, without another word from me, her lower lip drooped and began to slowly quiver. Seconds later, the tears were flowing. We both—she through her tears—laughed aloud. Here was a mother, wise in a worldly sense, accomplished in every way, totally in love with her baby and yet emotionally bereft!

SURPRISE: Postpartum Depression Can Happen with Dads Too

Q: Can dads experience postpartum depression?

A: Surprise! The answer is yes. Ten percent of men experience postpartum depression too. Financial stress, feeling like a third wheel, temporary loss of their sex life, a change in their relationship with their partners, an altered lifestyle, and sleep deprivation all contribute to their slumps. Others feel a sense of jealousy toward their child when they are required to share the attention of their partner with the baby.

Dad, if you think you may be experiencing postpartum depression, don't be afraid to seek out help and express the feelings you have. You are *not* weak or alone in your situation. Having a baby is one of the biggest experiences of a lifetime, bringing lots of drastic changes that are hard to adjust to. Getting the help you need at this time will allow you to be the best dad you can be to your new child.

Dads Continue to Be Important Beyond the Newborn Period!

The benefits of having an involved father are legion. Study after study demonstrates the value of having a dad who is responsive and actively participating in the lives of his children. In the biblical book of Malachi, it's considered a great blessing for a family and a culture when "a man's heart turns toward their children and the hearts of the children [turn] to their fathers."

Involved fathers during the newborn period and beyond enhance the quality of their children's lives in many ways: from cognitive, emotional, and social development to a sense of well-being, a decrease in negative child outcomes, and even physical health. Here are just some of the ways the presence of a father can positively impact a child.

Cognitive Development: Studies show that children with dads who are actively involved in their lives (measured by amounts of interaction, levels of play, and caregiving) are more cognitively competent at six months of age, scoring higher on the Bayley Scales of Infant and Toddler Development tests. Specifically:

- **At one year of age,** their developmental advanced prowess continues.
- **At three years of age,** they have higher IQs.
- **School-aged children** with involved daddies have better quantitative and verbal skills, score higher on achievement tests, and have higher grade point averages. They even *enjoy* school more!

Emotional Development: Infants whose dads are actively involved in their lives have a deeper sense of security, handle strange situations better, are more resilient in stressful situations, exhibit greater curiosity, and show more eagerness to explore their environments. These are all positive findings that bode well for these children.

Social Development: Fathers who are engaged with their children also produce offspring who are more socially developed. They demonstrate better social competence, social initiative, and social maturity, and they have a capacity to relate better with others. These children have more positive peer relations and tend to be more popular and liked by their peers.

Decrease in Negative Child Development Outcomes: Children with involved dads have reduced potential for future episodes of depression and sadness as well as reduced engagement in antisocial or adverse behaviors later in life, including substance abuse, delinquency, truancy, stealing, and lying.

Benefits for Physical Health: Children raised in a father-absent home are twice as likely to suffer from obesity, and infant mortality is twice as high too. "Present" dads also indirectly influence the health of their children by optimizing the health of mothers. Moms with supportive partners enjoy a greater sense of well-being and a more positive postpartum period than single mothers or mothers where the father is not involved at all. This translates into healthier children as well.

Stay-at-Home Dads and Paternal Leave

Aside from breastfeeding, men can learn the ropes of early childcare and do an amazing job. The number of families opting to have Daddy at home is increasing. These fathers who assume the role of caretaker reap the rewards of the job: they get to bond with their children and enjoy watching their young ones change daily in front of their eyes.

These are all reasons why a dad should take paternal leave if it is available to them. Dads play an important role throughout the newborn stage and beyond. Don't miss out on it! The experience and presence brings goodness to you, your baby, and Mommy too.

Moms and Dads Are Equal Players

Parents form a lovely, woven-together, complementing team. Like a teeter-totter, when one member of the team is down, the other is up, but if one goes missing, the whole program is thrown off. Moms and dads are *both* needed, *and you need each other* to raise a child successfully. And since children love both of their parents with equal intensity, "Dad time" is as important to them as "Mom time."

As we have seen, there are a slew of hormones that affect and prepare both moms and dads for the job of child raising. Yes, mothers are endowed with a greater share of these hormones and may thus have a natural advantage over the fathers, but dads, when your babies start fussing, you don't need to immediately hand them back to their mothers. Figure out how to comfort and help your child as handily as its mother. It can be done, and it is important that these skills be learned.

Raising children is a gigantic investment of time and energy, but if moms and dads do it together as a team, raising children is *fun!* And everyone wins, especially your baby.

So enjoy the experience of parenthood together as each parent plays a unique and critical role in the life of the child.

11

. . . . .

Oh, the Places You'll Go,
Where Your Children Take You

I recently attended a bar mitzvah where the grateful mother, while thanking the people who had come to witness her son read from the Torah, looked around the crowded room full of friends and family and made an insightful comment. With heartfelt gratitude and tears in her eyes, she reflected on the delights and joys her son had brought to her life, and then she added, "As I look around this room at all the wonderful people here today, I realize that my husband and I only knew 20 percent of you before our son was born."

It was a remarkable and profound statement.

What this mother was conveying with this thought was this: after Ryan, their son, had been born, their world had been rocked. The richness of their lives and their understanding and knowledge of the world had exploded, and contributing to that explosion for this family were the many new and interesting people who were now playing important roles in their lives.

Not only had Ryan's birth enriched them with happy and exciting family moments—guests would view a full panoply of their adventures in a slide show that was shown at a giant hotel bash later that night—but their son had brought many new and dear friends into their orbit as well.

The universe that they had previously known had enlarged.

Not only was she thankful, she was amazed!

New Friends and a New Universe

When children are born, they introduce us to the parallel universe of parenthood, a world that has always existed but is invisible to those without children. But as moms and dads are swallowed deeper and deeper into the parental experience, they enter and become intimately acquainted with a fresh, bustling, and dynamic new space filled with activity and noise—*lots* of noise—and color. It's the world of children.

Children, by their needs and their very nature, bring their parents to new places, and along the way, they also introduce them to many new friends.

There's a comfort in sharing experiences with people who are going through the same chaos and challenges that you are going through. These people become your friends, and many of these new friendships, germinated during the formative years of your young family, endure forever. We raise our children together with these other families and frequently find ourselves spending the rest of our lives intimately intertwined with them.

This is a good thing. Humans were never meant to raise children alone since by our nature, we are social creatures. We really do need each other, and here I am talking about a larger, more expansive "each other," like the extended family and a supportive society, to do the job well. Sharing and commiserating with others who are equally exhausted from colicky and sick babies binds us with these individuals with bonds that are strong and secure.

For many in our modern Western culture, however, intimacy and close interaction with the larger community is not the norm. We live our lives behind gates and doors and hedges that cut us off from our neighbors, and thus we create a cultural independence that was never meant to be. As John Medina, Ph.D., put it in his book *Brain Rules for Baby*, "Modern society does its level best to shred deep social connections."

Children help us break through these barriers and link us back to the community. So embrace this opportunity to connect and allow these new "parent friends" into your life. In doing so, you will find that they will become part of the matrix you establish to help navigate the beautiful new universe of parenthood. Raising children is incredibly rewarding when experienced alongside others swimming the same waters. Some of the dearest relationships my wife and I still value today were forged years ago during those early parenting days.

> *Nobody ever before asked the nuclear family to live all by itself in a box the way we do. With no relatives, no support, we've put [the family] in an impossible situation.*
>
> —MARGARET MEAD

Harrison and Pam

This is how things happened with our friends Harrison and Pam, whom we met at our small church in Santa Monica. Leslie and I already had our first son, Josh, when we met Pam, who was then pregnant with their first son, and Harrison, a young, aspiring attorney.

Shortly after our introduction, they had their first son, Daniel. We then added a girl, our daughter Noel, to the family. They soon followed and had a little girl named Lauren. Then we had yet *another* girl named Sarah, and—guess what?—they went out and had *another* girl too, whom they named Lindsey. We were still even. Three to three.

But it didn't stop there. We then had our second boy, whom we named Peter. Not long after, they had their second boy, a sweet fellow named Clayton. Then we added yet another beautiful daughter, Emily Rose, who was our fifth child.

It was like dueling banjos. Not to be outdone, they had their fifth child, a daughter whom they named Stephanie. Finally, we had our sixth and final baby, a cherubic little girl named Hannah Joy. But not to let the Hamiltons outdo them, Harrison and Pam had their sixth and final baby—another lovely girl named Kate. Six to six: boy, girl, girl, boy, girl, girl, in that order, for each family. We were even and, lest the contest continue into eternity, we agreed to a tie.

Our families were symmetric, but it was enough to make people dizzy. Between our two families, we had twelve kids, so when we went places together, we usually took over the place. We matched perfectly, and for the most part, so did our children.

This highly unique and fun coincidence led to a deep and enduring bond between our families. Through the years, we vacationed together, attended countless events together, and confided with Harrison and Pam the worries and the challenges we faced as parents raising six kids. Of all the people in the world, *they understood the challenge!*

When our children had their birthday parties, their kids were there. When I led medical mission teams to Africa with a couple of my children in tow, Harrison was my right-hand man with one or two of his children next to him. When Harry turned fifty, we traveled together as couples (we weren't taking twelve kids along on this trip!) to Italy and Israel to celebrate. When Pam's father, Poppy, passed away, we mourned and prayed together, and when our daughter Emily married our son-in-law Matt, Harrison presided over the wedding.

I could go on and on.

Enjoying life together with Harrison and Pam and their children has been one of the great blessings of our lives. Even today, Leslie and Pam take a weekly hike together in the local mountains while Harry and I set aside Saturday mornings for a weekly walk. While I tend to pontificate, his role is to poke me with his witty puns, keeping me humble and my feet securely planted on terra firma.

And all this happened because we started a family.

Close friends are truly life's treasure. Sometimes they know us better than we know ourselves. With gentle honesty, they are there to guide and support us, to share our laughter and our tears. Their presence reminds us that we are never really alone.

—ANONYMOUS

Friends for Life

Once a new baby starts developing inside the womb of a mother, it quickly becomes more and more difficult to hide the increasingly obvious baby bump. A mom's swollen tummy becomes a calling card to other parents-to-be. Like the proverbial birds of a feather, pregnant couples find each other and flock around each other to share this exciting experience.

Our Founding Fathers probably weren't thinking about pregnant women and their partners when they included the right to freedom of assembly in the Constitution, but they did understand the natural proclivity of individuals to find and enjoy being with their own, others going through the same season of life. Finding common ground with others and sharing the experience together is a good thing.

When Leslie was pregnant with Josh, we met several other pregnant couples (this was before we met Harrison and Pam) whom we grew very close to. It was an exciting time. After graduating from college, however, we moved to a different part of the state, and although we lost the everyday intimacy with those couples, we have managed to stay in touch and continue to regard these couples as dear friends.

Recently, we were at a wedding that a handful of these old friends also attended. Instantly, as if a time machine had transported us back in time, the warmth and delight of those early relationships that we cherished and remembered so fondly were rekindled in seconds. We had bonded during those early days of parenthood, and though we don't have the opportunity to see each other with the frequency we once did, the bond that was forged during those formative years has never faded.

Making Friends Doesn't Come Easy for All

While making new friends through the experience of parenting may come naturally to some, it may be more difficult for those who have unique circumstances. Perhaps you have recently moved to a new town or you're a frequently moving military family.

My advice to you is this: don't panic and don't worry! Your village of friends is out there for you too, though it may take some effort to find them. If you do find yourself struggling to find mommy or daddy friends to share your experiences with, here are a few ways you may be able to meet some.

- **Go to the Park:** Local parks are where children and parents congregate. It's neutral ground. Look for other parents with children the same age as yours, and engage them in conversation. Ask a question or two about their children and maybe even give them a compliment: "I love her curly hair!" or "He looks adorable in those overalls." If it feels natural, keep the conversation going. You will probably find something in common to talk about.

- **Check Facebook for Local Parenting Groups:** Do a quick Facebook search to see if there are any local parenting groups in your city. This is a great way to find other parents who share the same concerns that you have.

- **Attend Reading Time at the Library or Bookstore:** Check your local library or bookstore for story times. Since these are recurring, you will probably see the same mommies and daddies who bring their kids often, making it easy to build relationships.

- **Check Meetup.com for Local Playgroups:** Meetup.com is a handy website that allows anyone to form groups for people to gather around all sorts of shared interests, from knitting to hiking to cooking—and even parenting! You might be able to find a local playgroup this way where you can meet other parents and allow your kids to play together at the same time.

- **Find a Kid-Friendly Coffee Shop and Become a Regular:** Bigger cities often have wonderful coffee shops that offer play areas for small children and delicious drinks and snacks for everyone. If you become a regular at one of these places and bring your kiddos along, you will probably meet other regulars with kids too. Plus, who doesn't love a good cup of coffee and adult conversation after you've been engulfed in baby talk for so long?

- **Attend Church:** Religious institutions often have programs for parents and children. This is a good way to simultaneously teach your little one your faith and meet parents who share your faith as well. Church congregations tend by nature to be welcoming, which makes it all the easier.

SURPRISE: The friends your child chooses to play with will end up being your friends too, and, almost by definition, the parents of your child's friends will become your friends too.

Seek Out Kind Hearts

These new friendships you make are significant. Your children are going to be playing with your friends' children, and your friends' children are going to be playing with your children. The friends that your children choose to play with ultimately influence them in a big way, and it's an inescapable fact that *their* children will expose yours to the overall ethos of their families.

Find friends who have kind hearts—those dreamers, lovers, and poets who will love your children and teach them the same way you do. They're out there, and you'll find them if you look. They will become another facet of the bigger community that will enrich your lives. So choose wisely, keeping your radar on for moms and dads who share your ethics and values.

Old Friends and New

It's common to find that maintaining friendships with the people you spent time with *pre-baby* is difficult. Partly it's because going out with a baby is a bit more challenging than it was in your footloose past.

While this might come as a disappointment as some relationships wane, don't forget your old friends, and think of ways to creatively connect with them. Dinners out with your nonparent friends may not be possible with a baby in your arms, but brunches and dinners at your home may work. And never forget, we still have telephones, and a call to an old friend to simply catch up can be one of the kindest acts you do during a busy day.

And there is another reason to keep up with your nonparent friends. Who you were *before* you had children is part of your life's narrative. It's equally as important to remember who you were before you were a parent as it is to know where you are going now that you are a parent. Engaging and continuing to pal around with your old chums keeps those pre-parent days of your life living and relevant.

And finally, as the seasons of life change for all of us, many of these old friends, the ones you beat to the "baby party," get married and have children too. When this happens for them, these old friends tend to pop back into your life in a fresh and new way.

New Friends Are a Good Thing

The truth is, however, that the intensity of raising children causes individuals who are experiencing the same challenges to look for others and bond with them. So as you venture into this new pathway, your circle of friends will enlarge. In many cases, it'll be radically transformed, and you'll find yourselves hanging out with an entirely new group. Couples who have children when you have children become your new friends, and in many cases, they'll be together with you for years. This is your new cohort. Embrace them and they will embrace you. It turns out, you need one another to survive.

Yes, that's right, I mean *survive*, both while you have young children and beyond. Researchers have shown that people with strong friendships live healthier and longer lives. When you meet new people and develop friendships with them, your horizons expand; you learn new things, and this helps to keep your brain sharp, vital, and more open to new ideas.

Friends also bring happiness. A study published by *The British Journal of Psychology* in 2016 examined more than fifteen thousand respondents and found that people who had more social interactions with close friends were happier individuals. Having friends has also been shown to decrease blood pressure, diminish stress, and reduce the risk of depression—primarily because having someone else around looking out for you and watching your back brings comfort. This is especially true when parenting.

Another one of the great things about new parents connecting with and making friends with other parents is that when you know them well, *you've found someone you can trust to watch your child*—only at the cost of returning the favor. This isn't the sole reason for young couples to befriend one another, but in today's society, with our extended families living far away, many young parents simply don't have the convenience of an available grandparent or other family member who can babysit while Mom goes to the doctor or when both Mom and Dad get out for a quiet dinner. This is where close friends come in.

> *When you have kids, you do grow up. I have just started*
> *realizing it now—it changes the world, having children.*
>
> —DAVID BECKHAM

You Lead Your Children, but They Lead You Too!

Just when you think you're the one in charge, you'll find that your new baby is leading you to new places too. So get ready: that sweet little baby that you hold in your arms or even your unborn baby that you are waiting to meet, in addition to introducing you to lots of new friends, is also going to introduce you to new places that you never even knew existed, like ob-gyn offices filled with other women with big tummies, chaotic and insane pediatric offices crawling with screaming babies, lactation consultants' rooms laden with doodads and gizmos most guys have *never* laid eyes on before, stores filled with secondhand kids' clothes, and finally, the most baby-friendly coffee shops in town.

New parents with wee ones will also find that their children will cause them to become intimately familiar with the local parks, "Mommy and me" classes, infant swim classes, and baby ballet. And as they grow, your children will also engage you in other exciting activities. For example, when our daughters took a liking to and had an aptitude for volleyball, Leslie and I discovered yet another universe that we never knew existed. Girls' volleyball in Southern California is a *big deal*, and we got to experience it to the fullest.

Every weekend in Los Angeles, there are huge gymnasiums swarming to the brim with young girls playing volleyball. Inside these vast sport cathedrals, volleyballs, like launched missiles, fly at high speeds while crowds of sleepy parents cheer for their girls. The cacophony of these events defies description.

Who would have known?

Since our girls were into volleyball in a big way, we attended innumerable games and tournaments, had a wonderful time, and met lots of new friends along the way.

In addition to volleyball, we also discovered park-league basketball teams, Little League baseball, high school football, girls' gymnastics, ballet, violin lessons, and even cello camp—to name a few of the activities that our children were involved in.

The Adventures Never End

During our children's college years, we were introduced to still other exciting places. Because we chased our children to and fro, we got to explore historic Boston, tour Harvard Yard, walk along Chicago's exciting lakeside, revel in Wheaton College's tree-lined campus, drink lattes in character-filled Portland, Oregon, and finally, struggle to understand how anyone could ever get any studying done at Malibu's majestic, ocean-side Pepperdine campus.

And those are just some of the domestic locations our children "found" for us. They've also taken us to some of the far reaches of the earth. I must admit that this was partly our doing, because Leslie and I made it a mission to track our children down—to make sure all was well, mind you—whenever they did any semester-abroad programs. As a result, our children again took the lead and brought us to exotic places like Valparaiso, Chile, romantic Buenos Aires, ancient Jerusalem, staid Oxford, and rocking, rolling, and never-sleeping Salamanca, Spain.

Never a One-Way Street

It's never a one-way street when it comes to children. When they are born into our lives, they're the ones who are the neediest, but there is another counterintuitive truth also present.

Parents are needy too!

Young men and women who have been busy focusing their lives on building careers and fulfilling educational dreams now boast new titles: *Mommy* and *Daddy*. Having a baby causes people to look up from the cubicles that they've been inhabiting and see a new and broader vista: a panorama of life that includes a future and a legacy that must be wrestled with and established. For new parents, it's the proverbial (and much-needed) kick in the butt that human beings seem to need every so often.

The net effect is this: children help bring us to a place of greater maturity. They teach us things like patience and kindness and caring and selflessness, which we thought we already knew but really didn't. They shepherd us as much as we shepherd them and teach us things that some of us wouldn't have otherwise ever learned had children not been a part of our lives.

Finally, they bring us to both actual places and metaphorical places that we also would never have visited or known without their existence.

So as you give your energy, your time, and your lives to your sweet little ones during the first year, it's important that you also realize that a good portion of what you are doing for them *is indeed for your own good!* Yes, babies are impossibly helpless, but this is how the scheme works. It's through their fragile vulnerability that they give back to us.

And as you attend to their never-ending neediness, they will escort you to new joys, take you to new places, help you grow up, and, in the process, introduce you to new friends whom you wouldn't have ever known or met had it not been for your baby.

Yet another secret new parents uncover when babies come into their lives.

12

. . . . .

Resist the Allure of Screen Time

Secret #6: No Screens for the First Year of Your Child's Life

The world's first television station began broadcasting in 1928 from a General Electric laboratory facility in Schenectady, New York. The star of the show was a papier-mâché statue of Felix the Cat, rotating on a turntable. It was a humble beginning for a medium that would ultimately command our undivided attention and profoundly influence our culture.

From those early scratchy images that researchers broadcast between themselves, it was another twenty-five years before television entered American homes as a welcome balm to a world traumatized by a devastating war that had inflicted unimaginable death and untold pain.

The advent of television into American life began a torrid love affair that has never abated. Midcentury photographs of that era show well-dressed, happy families smiling as they gathered in elegant living rooms around colossal television cabinets with disproportionately small TV screens.

Those quaint scenes are far removed from the television we know today. Gone are those idyllic family gatherings around the television. Gone too is the benign content. Television today pours forth images of violence and superficiality. Crass, bratty, and vapid TV stars have replaced life-affirming characters like Andy Griffith and Lucy, who taught their viewers virtue, frugality, and modesty.

Much of today's television content undercuts traditional morality, and anyone—young or old—who watches television on a consistent basis will have its content soak into his or her psyche to some extent. This debasement of values is a challenge for our culture, but this isn't news. That has been a topic of conversation for the past several decades, and solutions continue to elude even the best thinkers.

What is news, however, is that television and an assortment of electronic screens have moved from the living room and are now, suddenly, *omnipresent*. The result of this ever-present availability of one form of screen or another means today's children are being exposed to screen time for longer and longer portions of their day.

The Ubiquity of Screens

For the parents of a less-than-one-year-old baby, the ever-present reality of televisions and electronic screens creates a never-ending sticky wicket. Some form of "blinking eye" is beckoning for our attention in nearly every home, restaurant, sports bar, and hospital room. *Gas stations* have even gotten into the act with screens entertaining us while we fuel up our cars. (Who would have ever thought that we needed to be entertained while we filled our cars with gasoline?) In fact, there's hardly a moment in our day when a smartphone, computer, or a touch pad to order our meal is outside our visual field.

Pediatrics offices are no exemption. Although we do our best in our office to be a screen-free zone, many parents import them like *contraband* into the office for their children to watch while they wait. And virtually every teenage patient that I have in my practice is head down, glued to their cell phones when I open the exam door.

I understand this. I spend entirely too much time looking down at my smartphone too.

Sometimes, however, these screens, in the context of me performing my duties as a physician, become an impossible distraction. On more than one occasion, I've instructed parents to turn down the volume of the video game their child is playing so we can communicate or, sometimes, to even listen to their child's heartbeat. With my teenage patients, I ask them to turn off their devices completely so I can see their faces and engage them in an actual, real-time, non-Skyped conversation.

The Power of Electronic Devices

For infants and young children, the hyperstimulation of electronic devices has been shown by several studies to have a negative effect on their cognitive and emotional development. Most of us, if asked to guess, would have intuited this outcome before the data proved it.

For concerned parents, countering this electronic media barrage requires a thought-out plan. It also calls for an assiduous, forward-thinking devotion to and protective love for their children. Some critics may characterize this overweening attempt to shield children from electronic screens as an arcane, reactionary plea for unrealistic simplicity. (Their argument is this: your children are going to have to deal with it sooner or later, so don't be so stiff.) I'd rather like to think of it as an appreciation for *tranquility* and as a proactive, tangible way to help make your kids smarter.

By the way, parents are not helpless. They are not at the mercy of these omnipresent interrupters as much as they think. The good news for moms and dads is this: every electronic device that engages you in mortal, hand-to-hand combat has an OFF button.

What's a Parent to Do?

In November 2011, the American Academy of Pediatrics (AAP) came out with recommendations regarding screen time for children under two years of age. As they had done in the past, they affirmed their recommendation that children during the first two years of life—a critical developmental period—should *avoid screen time completely.*

This recommendation for a total ban of screen time immediately produced controversy, and many detractors arose and deemed the AAP statement unreasonable and out of step with reality. Because of this pushback, the AAP reconsidered their policy and, more recently, came out with several more nuanced and personalized recommendations, which abandoned the one-size-fits-all guidelines previously proposed. These new, updated recommendations recognize the complexity of the new media, including interactive apps like Skype and FaceTime.

Some of the key points to the most recent AAP recommendations include:

- All screen time for children under eighteen months of age should be discouraged, except video chatting. Talking to grandparents via Skype is still a good thing!
- For children who are two years and older, screen time should be limited to one hour per day.
- Mealtimes should be screen-free, as well as the one hour before bedtime.

- Parents should view screen media with children aged eighteen to twenty-four months. The coauthor of the new AAP report calls this *structured joint attention*.
- Children under two years of age should not use screen media on their own.

It's Still Okay to Skype with Grandma!

Video chatting can be a wonderful way of connecting with family members, especially those who are far away. Skype and FaceTime can be used in the same way as telephone calls, and babies get the added benefit of seeing facial expressions.

Researcher Dr. Dimitri Christakis explained that apps like Skype and FaceTime are okay with young children because they are *interactive events* and take place in real time. These interactions are not passive moments but active communication. As he put it, "All screen-times are not the same."

What this AAP policy statement means for your less-than-one-year-old baby is still, however, very clear: *no screens allowed!*

Developmentally, babies don't *need* this input. They are obviously not mature enough to understand the content, but they are certainly distracted by our "talking boxes." But instead of being spellbound and hypnotized by the wiles of electronic gadgets, young children need to spend their days being stimulated in other ways.

What Happens When Infants Are Constantly Exposed to Electronic Screens?

There is good scientific evidence that supports these AAP recommendations. Several studies show that children exposed to screen time during the first couple of years are negatively impacted in various ways.

For starters, there is no compelling evidence that young children *learn* anything from early television watching in the first place, despite the claims that "educational programmers" make. Yes, there are some studies that show *some* benefits from high-quality educational programming for children who are *two years and older*, but steer clear of programming for your baby under one year of age.

And certainly, a screen will never teach like human interactions teach. Young children learn best through personal engagement—by touching, handling toys, and actively figuring out how things work. Hands-on, actual experiences are more valuable than passively watching and listening to someone else show them something.

Grandma Leslie and Luli Go Planting

Recently my wife, Leslie, took our granddaughter Luli into the yard to plant flowers. According to Leslie, Luli never missed a trick. Everything that Grandma Leslie did, Luli copied, even down to the placement of her feet while planting.

It was a delightful and unforgettable moment. Hands-on activities are how children learn about the world around them. This fun, outdoor chore was infinitely more valuable to the development of our granddaughter than her watching someone else plant flowers on television.

As children age, chronic early television watching in a home is linked to a reduction in language acquisition. Most likely this is due to a disruption of the parent-child interaction. Even if a child is not actively watching the television, *his parents are.* And this is where a big part of the problem lies. As the AAP report states, "It might be 'background media' to the child, but it is 'foreground media' to the parent."

John Medina, Ph.D., in his book *Brain Rules for Baby*, states that children are "aggressive learners," but goes on to explain that "human learning, in its most native state, is primarily a relational exercise." Engaged parents, those moms and dads who speak with and interact with their children daily, are helping to grow smart brains.

Children Learn Best from Live Interaction

So even if children are *not* watching the television themselves, their parents are being distracted from interacting with them, and as a secondary phenomenon, the richness of communication between the parent and the child erodes. Less interaction, language-wise, between parent and child means baby is hearing fewer words in any given day, and the end result of this kind of word-starved environment for the baby is an impoverished and scant vocabulary later.

There are children who literally hear *millions* more words during their early childhood years because their parents spoke to them more. This makes a big difference in their verbal skills when it comes time for formal schooling, because a rich spoken language proceeds the successful mastery of written language. Children who grow up in homes with omnipresent televisions are at risk for having delayed cognitive development and reading comprehension challenges.

Dr. Dimitri Christakis studied "audible television" in a home and its association with infant vocalizations and adult conversation. He and his coworkers found that "having a television on was associated with significant reductions in discernible parental word counts, child vocalizations, and 'conversational turns' for children 2 to 48 months of age." In other words, when the TV is on, parents are preoccupied and not interacting with their children.

This should not come as a surprise. People who watch TV are

concentrating on what is happening on the screen. When it comes to television viewing, it's almost impossible to multitask. Have you ever tried to have a conversation with someone who is engrossed in the evening news? And how is it possible to have rich interaction with the infant at your feet when there's a football game airing? Dr. Christakis's research team found that word counts decreased significantly during television watching times by up to five hundred to one thousand words per hour of television watching time. This means that parents who habitually watch television, when their children are young, are depriving them of *thousands* of audible words daily. We all learned that "sticks and stones may break my bones, but words will never hurt me." That cute little adage may or may not be necessarily true, but one thing is for sure: *no words* really do hurt.

The Christakis paper concluded, "Having a television on within earshot of young children diminishes their exposure to adult words, their own vocalizations, and the conversational turns in which they engage."

Ouch!

Media Overuse

The magnitude of media watching cannot be overstated. Earlier AAP reports noted that nearly 40 percent of families with young children have televisions on *all the time*, and a shocking 20 percent of children—babies who are less than *one year* of age—have televisions in their rooms. Even though babies are not necessarily watching these screens, this background media—sometimes called *secondhand television*, like secondhand smoke—has a negative effect on a child's development.

Equally sobering is research that shows that for *every hour* of media programming a child watches per day in the first three years increases a child's odds of manifesting attention deficit hyperactive disorder *by 10 percent* when assessed for ADHD at seven years of age. What that means is this: children who watched an average of one hour per day of television during the first three, developmentally critical years of their lives were shown to have a 10 percent chance of having ADHD at seven years of age. And it went up from there. Children who watched an average of two hours of media entertainment manifested ADHD symptoms at a rate of 20 percent, and those sad children who watched an average of three hours of television a day during those critical years had a shocking 30 percent chance of having ADHD at seven.

> *Childhood itself is disappearing into the bewitching embrace of technology.*
> —MEGHAN COX GURDON, ESSAYIST, JOURNALIST, AND
> CHILDREN'S BOOK REVIEWER FOR *THE WALL STREET JOURNAL*

Healthy Distraction for Your Children

There comes a moment in every parent's day when he or she needs his or her own time out—to sit for a few minutes, take a shower, or read a newspaper. Screens are most often the distraction of choice for babies at those times, but here are some other options.

- Play audiobooks: Even for young babies, audiobooks can help with language acquisition and development. Set up a space where your baby can play with blocks or soft toys in safety while the story is read.
- Put some music on: Babies and young children love tunes and a beat, so play them nursery rhymes, soft jazz, stirring orchestral works—something bright and serene.
- Hand them a book: Sure, babies are a little young to read for themselves, but they will be entranced by flipping the pages and looking at the pictures in a soft book or board book.

It Doesn't Stop There—More Negative Effects

As if the points above aren't enough, there are several other ways having a television on around your child will negatively affect him. It is important for you as a parent to be aware of all the ways something so seemingly harmless can have such a disagreeable impact on your tiny developing, growing, and changing baby. Here are three more reasons to turn off the tube.

1. High Levels of Television Watching Diminish Active Play

Active play is defined as time when a child is physically doing something. This physical activity can be as simple as grabbing things, chewing on objects, rolling over, attempting to crawl, or pulling up to a stand. According to the AAP, this "unstructured playtime is critical to learning problem-solving skills and fostering creativity."

These are the moments that children are actively engaged in heeding and fulfilling that inner blueprint that keeps a child on that aggressive, never-ending quest to learn and grow. But television can exert such a powerful control on a baby's attention (and older children, teens, and adults too) that it can quench and subtract from the time that children engage in active play.

The Three Rules of Stamm for Babies and Television

Early brain developmental expert and author of the book *Bright from the Start,* Dr. Jill Stamm has developed three simple rules for screen use in your own home:

- No screens in your child's bedroom
- No screen in the car
- Turn off the television completely when you are playing with your baby in the living or family room

2. Media Watching Diminishes the Opportunity for Downtime

Infants and children also need downtime, a time during the day when they are *not* being stimulated. These quiet, unstructured, "unplugged" moments allow young infants an opportunity to accomplish tasks and learn new things with minimal adult intervention. It's during these downtime moments that babies look around and explore their environment. They make choices of which toy *they want* to grab, as opposed to having one handed to them. They touch and feel items and see how they work. And, almost as important, they learn how to entertain themselves.

Downtime also allows infants the freedom to develop a sense of independence. They even learn that being alone can be fun. This alone, doing-nothing time is frequently heard (and sometimes seen) by parents in the early morning when babies awaken. Most children don't wake up to their day crying. Rather, when babies awaken, before they call out to their mothers, they frequently move about their cribs, babble to themselves, discover their feet, reach for their mobiles, and play quietly with their toys. This is downtime at its best and truly delightful for parents to see and hear.

Babies are adorable, and it's natural for family members and visitors to want to occupy them in fun activities like reading to them, swinging them, and playing with them on the floor. Don't get me wrong—these are all wonderful things to do with your babies, but there is something to be said for letting babies *just be*. In other words, children don't always need external stimulation because they are quite capable of entertaining themselves if they are given the opportunity.

Some parents never get this memo. There are a lot of overstimulated children out there, those poor souls who are never allowed to have any quiet or reflective moments. Child psychologist Dr. Vicki Panaccione has studied these overstimulated children and has found that they exhibit higher levels of anxiety "because there is so much coming at them and their little nervous systems can only handle so much." The omnipresent electronic screens contribute much to this overstimulation.

And although there is an entire industry of "baby-friendly" learning tools like books, puzzles, specialized toys, CDs, and videos, new parents should not be misled into thinking that children—especially young babies—need these tools to develop normally. Sometimes less is more.

So relax and remember that babies need quiet time to rest their brains and their bodies. Enjoy the silence, and don't let television and computer screens rob them of these unstructured moments. Know too that these quiet moments are exactly what your babies need to allow their fresh imaginations and nascent creativity to flourish.

3. Television Disrupts Sleep Patterns

Darcy Thompson, M.D., MPH, studied sleep schedules in children who regularly watched TV and found that "television viewing among infants and toddlers is associated with irregular sleep schedules." It is not completely clear why this is so, but research suggests that the bright light of the television before sleep affects the sleep-wake cycle by suppressing the release of melatonin. Melatonin is a naturally occurring hormone made in the pineal gland. It is released about 90–120 minutes before a person's usual bedtime, and it helps humans (and other animals as well) synchronize their circadian rhythms, particularly sleep cycles. Bright lights suppress the release of melatonin and thus make sleep less possible.

Another theory of why television affects young children's sleep cycles relates to the content of the material children see. In young infants, who clearly do not understand the nature of what they see, this argument is less compelling, but they do hear noises and see images. These stimuli can have a negative effect on relaxation, which is necessary for sleep to occur.

Get the Facts: Babies, Toddlers, and TV Today

- About 90 percent of parents admit that their children younger than two years of age routinely watch some form of electronic media (TV, videos, web-based programming, CDs, DVDs, iPads).
- By three years of age, 30 percent of children have televisions in their rooms.
- Many parents use TV as a babysitter or "peacekeeper" and regard it as a safe activity for their children when they are preparing a meal, doing household chores, showering, or getting ready for work.
- Parents are happier and feel better when their children watch educational TV programs.
- Parents who believe that educational television is "very important for healthy development" are twice as likely to have the TV on "all or most of the time."
- On average, children younger than two years of age watch televised programs one to two hours per day.
- At least 14 percent of children aged six to twenty-three months watch two or more hours of media daily.

Children who live in lower-socioeconomic-status homes and children with mothers having less than a high school education are spending more time in front of a screen daily than their wealthier counterparts. Naomi Schaefer Riley wrote in a 2016 *Wall Street Journal* article, "What no one tells low-income families is this: The real digital divide is between parents who realize the harmful effects of technology on their children and try to limit them, and those who don't. It's the difference between parents

> buying wooden blocks this Christmas and those racking up more credit-card debt to buy their child a LeapPad."
>
> Children who live in households with "heavy media use" (homes where the television is on all or most of the time) spend 25–38 percent less time being read to (or reading) than other children. They also have a lower level of reading abilities when compared to homes with "low media use."

Final Thoughts About the Boob Tube

Walking through our neighborhood in the evening hours is an education. I'm not spying on anyone, but it is impossible not to notice the living rooms illuminated with the glow of televisions.

During these quiet strolls, I can't help but notice that most houses have televisions blazing with gigantic screens that sometimes cover entire walls. The high-definition clarity is lifelike, and the color is perfect. Gone are the green faces and orange hair of yesteryear's early color televisions.

During some of these evening strolls, I confess that I sometimes find myself stopping, without even being aware of what I am doing, and watching from the sidewalk, through my neighbor's window, a crazy gunfight or a wild chase scene that's playing on the wall-to-wall television.

I know I look like a stalker or some sort of Peeping Tom, but who can avoid being thoroughly mesmerized? I don't berate myself too much when this happens because I blame my curiosity on human nature. I am one of us, and humans crave action and excitement.

But there's a lesson here. If adults are so entranced with this technology, think for a moment about your young infants. They're going to be enthralled too. And that's exactly what happens! And by the way, there is an army of media technocrats, lots of very smart guys and gals working in New York City, who have designed it to be just so.

But make your babies wait!

They *need* to wait because during the first year of life, their little brains are maturing at lightning speed and they need to stay focused. Flashing screen images distract them from their task.

Parents appreciate this neuronal maturation indirectly as they tick off their children's developmental milestones.

Smile at Mommy, check.

Roll over from tummy to back, check.

Reach out and grab a rattle, check.

These predictable developmental milestones that parents see happening before their eyes are evidence of their babies' brains coming online. We shouldn't allow any interference with this process. Viewing of electronic media during infancy, especially when it is excessive, pushes the Pause button in your child's brain. Rather than being an active learner, your baby becomes a passive watcher.

There are only so many hours in one day, and there are only 365 days in your baby's most valuable first year. Every minute that a child dedicates to watching a screen steals from her a minute that she could be doing something more enriching and productive.

For those rare individuals who are concerned that their children will fall behind in this digital age without early exposure, understand that research shows the direct opposite results. More likely than not, your child is going to have a lifetime of screen time, either at her job or through entertainment. There is no need to fret: she will get her fill.

But not now.

Let your tender baby nestle in the warm, loving cocoon of infancy that you have created for her, sheltered far away from the babble and the blare of the electronic-screen storm.

And enjoy together each moment of these early, simple days—because they are short.

13

. . . . .

Travel Far and Wide

SURPRISE: The world is *still* your oyster!

My wife and I were once visiting Montenegro, a small country on the Dalmatian coast. While there, I took a hike on an arduous but lovely trail that looked out over the Adriatic Sea. During my trek, I occasioned to meet a young couple with two children coming the other way. One of their children, a young girl, was tucked comfortably into an infant carrier on her father's back while the other, a three- or four-year-old boy, dutifully shuffled along between his parents.

I was somewhat amazed to find this young couple and their children on this rather difficult trail. As I watched them pass, coaching and encouraging their son along, I could see that they were having a grand time doing what a lot of other people would have written off as being impossible . . . and even a bit crazy.

But there they were, enjoying a fantastic hike with an unparalleled vista. After they passed, I turned and took a second look at them and thought, *Bravo to you two! You guys are brave souls, and you're living life to its fullest.*

The Joy of Doing Crazy Things

Traveling with young children is one of the things lots of people have placed into the "impossible" category.

But it's not!

In fact, it is the very opposite.

And the first year of life is *exactly* the right time to do it.

> **SURPRISE:** Young babies travel well!

As a general statement, babies under one year of age are grand travelers. Of course, there are exceptions. I've certainly heard my share of travel horror stories (and don't hate on me if things go awry for you), but young children, especially young babies during the first few months of life—before they are crawling or starting to walk—travel much better than people think.

Infants find the roar of jet engines and the sound of a car on the road soothing. Even the bounce of airplane turbulence (which still fills me with terror) or the rocking of a boat or train (which induces motion sickness in many) provides comfort to a young child. They take it all in stride and, as the saying goes, they sleep like babies! So don't let details or trivialities keep you from grand adventures or from beloved family members who are only an airline flight or a road trip away.

You've Got an Obligation to Show Off Your Baby

One major reason why travel during the first year is important is family. Once baby has arrived, new parents have an obligation to show off their baby to their family and other dear friends. These are the same people who have been cheering for you and praying for you— and your baby—from the moment they learned you were pregnant. So introducing your newborn to these caring souls is your reciprocal act of loving-kindness. One of the true delights of becoming a new parent is introducing, for the first time, your newborn to family and friends.

In sharing your baby with your friends and family, you will vicariously appreciate the heartwarming joy that comes from watching *others* take delight in your child. People adore babies! When you bring your infant to visit the people in your life who love you the most, you are giving them a tangible opportunity to participate in the thrill that new life brings.

This is especially true for relatives or friends who are suffering from illnesses or other difficult situations. Babies light up every room they enter. They also bring hope, healing, and unutterable pleasure. The late Paul Kalanithi, M.D., in his book *When Breath Becomes Air*, described the aura that hovered over his newborn daughter as "a brightening newness [that] surrounded her."

My father-in-law was a very ill man during the final weeks and months of his life. When he learned of Leslie's pregnancy, there is little doubt in my mind that he mustered all the willpower he had to stay alive to meet his firstborn grandchild. When Josh was born and we were able to bring him to visit his grandfather, my father-in-law's suffering momentarily abated, and his face brightened with a weak smile. These were tender and unforgettable moments that we will never forget. In the darkest time imaginable, our newborn son brought his grandfather a glimmer of light and hope. The memories of the comfort that our infant son Josh brought to his grandpa Gene during those dark moments still bring solace and joy to both Leslie and me.

Take Baby on Your Business Trips Too

Okay, maybe I've convinced you to take your babies on your vacations and to also introduce them to your families. After all, when you think about it, it's tough to leave them behind. But when I recommend to my new moms and dads to put your babies in your back pocket and take them wherever you go, I'm including having them travel with you on your business trips too.

I know that this sounds a bit insane for busy professionals, but hear me out.

An African Observation

During my travels to Africa, I have taken note that the African woman is a busy individual. Not only is she found working in the fields along the roads, she's in the marketplace bartering and you'll find her riding on the crowded buses in the city and throughout the country.

For the African woman with a child, there is no difference that I can discern in the activities that she performs versus African women without children. This is because working women in Africa include their children in *all the tasks of everyday life*. Securely strapped to the backs of their mothers and thus having no choice in the matter, babies accompany their mothers wherever they go. The seemingly impossible chasm of being working mothers that American women straddle is seamless in Africa. Working African women don't skip a beat when they have babies.

Back Home in America

I have never recommended that Americans adopt all the traditions and ways of Africa. I have traveled to the continent enough times that I am no longer enchanted or romanced as I once was by all things African. The residents of Africa, like all peoples around the world, face their own unique challenges. That said, there are lessons Western women can learn from the ways African women include their children in all that they do.

When one becomes a parent, he or she enters a different dimension of life. Having a baby and caring for him or her isn't a babysitting gig. He or she is your *son* or *daughter* and the child should (and needs to be) integrated into the *total you*, and this includes all that *you do*—including your work, which includes your business travels.

This paradigm of caring for your child *all the time*, even during work responsibilities, is a different way of thinking for most Western parents. I understand this, but this notion isn't a foreign concept throughout most of the world, especially during the child's critical first months of life. This is where we can learn from the Africans.

Keeping babies with their mothers not only calms and brings mothers great peace and contentment, being close to their mothers early on is particularly beneficial for babies. Just as mothers intensely bond with their children, babies too *intensely bond with their mothers*. So separations—even seemingly brief separations—are difficult for everyone, but they're particularly difficult for young children.

One reason for this is because babies mark time differently from the way adults do. A busy, event-filled half day of work for an adult, which so quickly passes, can feel like an eternity for a baby. There's a reason why older children badger their parents with repeated "Are we there yet?" queries when traveling. And remember how hard it was for you to wait for summer vacation when you were a kid? For children less than one year of age, time moves even more slowly. Even a short, overnight business trip for Mommy represents a forever interval for a young babe, unless Mommy is surrounded by a strong support team which includes a deeply involved Daddy.

Another compelling reason for moms, especially for moms who are breastfeeding, to bring their babies with them is because *it's very difficult to find qualified and reliable people to care for children while they are away.* Unless one has a stay-at-home partner, a ready-and-willing grandmother, or a live-in nanny—*someone who can be trusted completely*—finding childcare for a young baby isn't easy. And this doesn't consider the logistical nightmare breastfeeding moms face when they have to pump their breasts and store their milk while on the road.

Finally, getting these things in order at home can also be expensive. Sometimes it's *cheaper* just to bring your baby (they fly free when they are young), buy a ticket for Grandma, Grandpa, babysitter, or nanny, and bring childcare *with* you.

So if it's at all possible, make it easier on yourself and your baby, and bring him with you during your travels—even your business travels—at least during the first year. This will require a touch of creativity and ingenuity, but when parents embrace the notion of having their young children accompany them *all the times*, the details work out.

Companies Who Are Getting It Right

Some employers recognize the value of easing business travel for new mothers and, as a result, are making it easier for moms to bring their children with them on business trips. One New

York–based investment firm, KKR, pays for nannies and infants to accompany mothers on their business-related travels during their babies' first year. This is a laudable decision. Smart companies who want to keep their talented and productive women executives in the firm (and very, very happy too) should consider similar benefits.

The glass ceiling will shatter for women when they participate in boardrooms that acknowledge all aspects of being women, which includes recognizing and embracing the fact that some women are mothers and mothering is a vital job too.

But even if your company doesn't provide such rich benefits, do whatever *you can do* to keep your child at your side during his or her first year. Even if your trip is all business, having your baby within reach or down the hall in a hotel room with a baby-sitter will curb much of the anxiety traveling mothers experience. And believe it or not, having your baby close at hand will make you and your travels much more enjoyable and even more productive.

A Family Who Grooved Together

One of the fathers in my practice was a professional musician who had a lot of kids and an *amazing* wife. Doing what he did for a living required him to spend weeks, even months on the road. But he did it right! When he was on the road, so was his family. His wife and kids traveled with him across the country and around the world. They are a remarkable family and, in my opinion, have some of the most winsome and well-adjusted kids I have ever known.

Five Simple Tips When Traveling with Babies

Before parents take the leap and travel with their children, they need to look ahead and make provisions. Here are five recommendations to consider when one of your traveling partners is a baby.

1. Don't fly with children under two months of age. By two months of age, babies who are getting their routine vaccinations on the recommended schedule will have received the first round of protective dosages of several immunizations. At this point in time, it's okay to take them along on commercial flights. *However, one note of caution:* if it's midwinter and the nation is amid an influenza epidemic, I recommend a delay in your plans for two reasons. First, young children who contract influenza get very sick, and second, pediatricians don't vaccinate children against influenza until six months of age. As young unvaccinated infants, they are more susceptible to infection.

For families who are taking a road trip, it's okay to travel with your children from the very start. Just remember that young infants, those under one month of age, have naive, untested immune systems. They also will not have received the first round of protective immunizations, so traveling families who are driving should employ great caution before taking their less-than-one-month-old child into public places like restaurants.

2. Go to one place at a time and stay there for a while. When you travel with a young baby, your trip should not be the "if this is Tuesday, this must be Belgium" kind of tour. Nor do you want it to be! Let's be perfectly honest about it: traveling with children is a different experience from any traveling you have ever done before. So when babies are a part of the equation, hopping from place to place in rapid succession will be less gratifying than ever before.

Instead, go to one place, unpack, and enjoy the view before moving on. This will allow your child to adjust to the new environment (and possibly a new time zone) before you explore your next destination.

Renting cabins, apartments, or houses is also a better bet for young families than hotels. The cost of renting self-contained accommodations over an extended time is more affordable than hotels. This arrangement also allows families more flexibility in food preparation and usually provides more space for you to spread out and for your child to explore.

3. Bring a minimum of things with you. Half the challenge of traveling with young children is the amount of stuff you must bring to care for them. For travelers who pride themselves in bringing the absolute minimum, the abundance of essential baby gear—diapers, diaper bags, car seats, blankets, and toys—will prove to be a vexation. You can still be a minimalist, but it will require a different game plan. (See box below.)

4. If possible, fly direct. Flying to London from Los Angeles via Albuquerque and Chicago is okay if you are a teenager heading to England for the summer. It's a totally different experience if you have a three-month-old child in tow. So, if possible, take direct flights.

Yes, one individual direct flight may be longer, but when the plane touches down, you're there. That isn't true when you have connections to make. Just getting from one plane to another in a busy airport with a babe in your arms can be daunting.

5. Invest in travel insurance. One never knows what tomorrow may bring. Travel insurance when trekking with children is always a good idea. If there is a reason to return home quickly, travel insurance will cover the cost of emergency transport back to your home, which is otherwise extremely expensive.

Traveling Light the Easy Way

When traveling with babies, the temptation is to pack for every possible contingency. The result? Bulging luggage and unwanted stress.

- Pack for most likely scenarios, not improbable disasters.
- Plan to wash clothes as you go. Better to take laundry detergent than superfluous changes of clothes.
- Choose the miniature, most compact version for things like strollers, toiletries, and diaper bags.
- Buy supplies as you go. You'll be able to purchase diapers and most other baby products almost anyplace you travel to.

Flying with Children

Today's commercial airlines are reliable, have exceedingly well-built aircraft, and are safer than any other form of transportation. Air travel is ten times safer, for example, than train travel. And the good news for traveling parents is that there are no special travel restrictions that apply to infants and children, except for those with rare medical conditions like cardiac or pulmonary illnesses. This means parents can take their children with them *anywhere* and *everywhere* airplanes fly.

Airplane Health

The fear of getting an infection on a flight is a concern I frequently hear from traveling families. Because of the proximity of other passengers, limited ventilation, and the impracticality of the airlines to screen for illness, airborne sicknesses can indeed spread person-to-person on airplanes.

But it's important also not to *overstate* the risks of flying. The risk of getting sick from airborne illnesses during a flight is *no different from* the risk of getting sick on buses or trains. Modern airplanes are also equipped with high-efficiency, sophisticated air filters that remove particles in the air. These filters effectively eliminate 99.9 percent of bacteria and viruses, which renders the air in an airplane equivalent to fresh air. Newer jets exchange their cabin air fifteen to twenty times per hour. This is more than the average home (five times per hour) or office building (twelve times per hour). Airflow on airplanes is also directed vertically, from top to bottom, not horizontally, the direction of airflow more likely to transmit infections.

Travel Safety

Besides airline safety, when you're a parent traveling with children, you are forced to consider lots of other what-ifs that most people prefer *not* thinking about. All kinds of things can and do go wrong when you are traveling whether you have a baby with you or not, but traveling parents with babies must plan for even more than the usual possibilities.

Here are five pearls that will help you increase the overall safety, success, and pleasure of your travels with your young child.

1. Bring a car seat for your baby. Motor vehicle accidents are the leading cause of injury and even death in children who travel, especially for those traveling abroad. Road conditions, congested roadways, and foolhardy drivers are to blame for these statistics.

In the United States, the law requires children who weigh fewer than forty pounds to be restrained. This is a matter of common sense. For those families traveling in foreign countries, however, where child restraint is not mandatory, parents should not be beguiled by lax safety laws. Bring a car seat with you, and secure your child in it in the middle of the back seat of the vehicle you are traveling in.

2. Rent a car with seat belts. Another related consideration for parents is seat belts. Some foreign countries—especially in the Third World—do not have seat belt laws, which means they may or may not be found in the taxis you hail. So even if you have carried a bulky and awkward car seat across an ocean or two, there may not be a seat belt to secure it in the taxi you're riding in.

This can be a big problem because the way some taxi drivers drive will cause you to squirm, especially if you have an unsecured baby on your lap. (By the way, whether traveling with a baby or not, if you think your driver is taking unnecessary risks, tell him to slow down! Don't be afraid to speak up.)

Savvy and well-traveled parents solve this car seat/seat belt taxi dilemma by renting a car with seat belts while visiting abroad.

3. If you do rent a car, don't drive long distances at night in foreign countries. Getting around a city at night is one thing, but driving from city to city through the countryside during evening and night hours is not advised. Road conditions vary widely, and prudence requires that you only drive when conditions are optimal.

4. Bring a small first-aid kit. Your less-than-one-year-old baby will probably not be getting too many scrapes or cuts while abroad, but babies do have fevers, diaper rashes, superficial skin infections, irritations, and diarrhea. Your first-aid kit should include a thermometer, liquid Tylenol, gas drops, saline drops for stuffy noses, diaper rash creams, Benadryl for allergies, oral rehydration solution packets for diarrhea, and some basic antibiotics that you can obtain from your pediatrician before your travels, like antibiotic eye drops for pinkeye and mupirocin (Bactroban) for superficial skin infections.

5. Prevent sunburn with hats, clothing, and sunscreen. Babies in the first tender months of their lives should be protected from too much direct sunlight. Excess ultraviolet radiation causes skin damage that is cumulative over a lifetime, so when your child is outside, apply a sunblock of SPF 50 to his skin.

Pediatricians do not routinely recommend sunblock for children under six months of age, but if parents find themselves with their less-than-six-month-old child outside with lots of sun exposure, a block can be applied. Before application, however, place a small test patch on the abdomen. If there is no reaction within thirty minutes, sunblock can then be applied more liberally to other areas of the body. Remember too that sunblock needs to be reapplied every two to three hours to maintain its effectiveness.

Clothing is useful to protect your baby from the sun too. Long-sleeved, tightly meshed UV-protective rash guards, along with sun hats, also keep children sun safe.

Preventing Infection While on the Road

There are a lot of little bugs lurking in this world. They're here at home, and you will find them out there, wherever you are going. The problem is, the microorganisms you encounter in the places you are going are often different from the ones that we live with at home. This means moms and dads must look ahead and prepare.

Effectively Treating Sunburn

Follow these steps to help heal your baby's sunburn:

1. Get out of the sun and rehydrate your child.
2. Cool the skin either by bathing in cool water or sponging the skin with cool towels. Do not use ice packs.
3. Put your baby in an oatmeal bath. Place two cups of oatmeal into a sock and drop it into a cool bath. Oatmeal has natural anti-inflammatory properties that will help ease any pain and discomfort.
4. Soak a washcloth in cold milk and place it on the burned skin. Milk is rich in proteins that have anti-inflammatory benefits.
5. Use soothing creams and lotions that contain ingredients like aloe vera, arnica, calendula flower, and coconut oil to help heal and moisturize skin, relieving any discomfort.
6. Stay out of the sun until the sunburn heals completely.

For sunburn pain, ibuprofen is the drug of choice.

Our job as parents is to do our best to keep these infectious (and dangerous) organisms away from our children. Fortunately, with the progress medicine has made over the past many years, we have tools to fight back.

Here is my short list of four simple recommendations parents should employ before they travel, both domestically and abroad, to avoid infection.

1. Immunizations: One of the most proven and effective ways to keep your children healthy is to immunize them. Pediatricians spend a considerable portion of our time encouraging moms and dads to immunize their children in a timely way, but for those parents traveling with young children, these recommendations take on a greater level of significance. The bottom line is this: your children should be up to date with all their vaccinations before you travel. When a family is traveling out of the country or taking a trip that will require an airline flight, the importance of this recommendation increases.

Airports, bus stations, and train stations are filled with people. As travel becomes more accessible and less expensive, people from all parts of the world are awakening to the joys of travel, and the number of people on the move is staggering. Like never before, we live in a highly connected, integrated world. In 2017, according to the International Air Transport Association, more than 4.1 billion individual journeys were taken on airplanes. This number doesn't include the billions upon billions of journeys people took on buses, trains, and boats, or in their cars.

So what does this explosion in worldwide travel mean to you and your family? Simply this: traveling will put you and your child in direct contact with a vast panoply of people. Since person-to-person transmission is one of the most common ways diseases spread, the potential for your child being exposed to disease increases. When you are traveling through a busy international airport, some of the people standing next to your family at the gate have exotic viruses and bacteria growing *in* them or *on* them.

I'm not sharing this with you to induce paranoia or keep families bottled up as shut-ins at home, but this is the reason vaccinations are important. Pediatricians routinely tell parents to immunize their children so their lovely offspring will be protected from these novel and pathogenic organisms. (And by the way, some of the people carrying those exotic bacteria and bizarre viruses in and on their bodies are your friends and neighbors. They take their children to the same parks that you do, shop at the grocery store down the street, and go to your church.)

2. Diarrhea Prevention: Infectious gastroenteritis is the most common travel-related illness that affects children. Since babies are small, they can experience dehydration more readily than adults. Therefore, diarrhea prevention needs to be an important consideration for parents traveling with small children.

Breastfeeding is pure and simple, so young babies who are breastfeeding should continue to do so, as this is the best way to prevent gastrointestinal illnesses in young children. With slightly older children, particularly that teething five-month-old baby, the six-month-old who has started on solid foods, and the nine-month-old child who has begun to crawl, scrupulous care must be taken in terms of what they put into their mouths, what they eat, and what they drink.

Preventing Diarrheal Disease in Children

- Water given to children should be disinfected by being boiled or chemically treated. Bottled water is the best to ensure sterility.
- Food given to children should be thoroughly cooked.
- Fresh fruits should be peeled before they are eaten.
- Care should be taken to hand-wash and clean bottles, pacifiers, teething rings, and toys that fall to the ground.
- For short trips, parents may consider bringing food from home in their luggage.

3. Protection from Mosquitoes, Ticks, and Fleas: Avoiding mosquito, tick, and flea bites has always been a paramount goal of travelers due to the serious diseases that they carry. The diseases carried by mosquitoes alone include Zika, malaria, dengue, chikungunya, yellow fever, and West Nile virus, to name just a few. Mosquito bite prevention is therefore an important goal in areas of the world where these diseases are present.

Protecting Your Baby from Insects

Q: How can I protect my baby from mosquitoes, ticks, and fleas?
A: There are several ways that parents can keep their children free of mosquito, tick, and flea bites during their travels.

- Keep your baby indoors during the early evening hours. Early evening is when mosquitoes feed, so this is the time to keep your children out of harm's way. (Some mosquitoes are also active during the day, so keeping your child protected from mosquitoes during the day is likewise important.)
- Keep your baby in long-sleeved clothing and socks when outside.
- Use treated mosquito netting over strollers and over cribs during nap and night hours. Overhead fans impede mosquitoes' ability to hover and land.
- Repellents can be applied to clothing and bed netting. Permethrin can be used and is active even after several washings of clothes. Permethrin should *not,* however, be applied to the skin.
- Skin repellents can be used, such as oil of lemon eucalyptus (OLE), picaridin, para-menthane-3,8-diol (PMD), and DEET. These repellants are helpful to use on your children when they are outside. When children return indoors, their skin should be washed clean from these repellents. Skin repellents should not be applied over cuts, open wounds, or skin rashes. Avoid putting repellent in or near children's eyes and mouths—and since children put their hands in their mouths and rub their eyes frequently, anti-mosquito repellents are *not* recommended for children's hands.

Q: Should I use DEET repellants if my child is younger than two months?
A: Children under two months should *not* have DEET applied to their skin.

Q: What percentage should the DEET product be that I use on my infant?
A: The standard recommendation is to use a repellent with *no more than* 30 percent DEET on children over two months of age.

Malaria Prevention

Malaria is one of the most serious, life-threatening diseases that afflicts children traveling internationally. If you are going to areas where malaria is prevalent, you need to take special precautions. Find out about areas of malaria by checking the Centers for Disease Control and Prevention's website (www.cdc.gov).

4. Infections from Soil Contact: Babies during the second half of their first year begin to roll over, scoot, crawl, and even walk. So in getting around, they tend to spend more of their waking hours closer to the ground and, hence, in harm's way from microorganisms that live in the soil. In your home, you can control the cleanliness of their environment, but in far-flung vacation spots, you won't get to have that kind of control. The sands of those foreign beaches and the dirt of distant parks are alive with all sorts of organisms, including parasites like hookworm, ascaris, and visceral larva migrans. You don't need to remember the names of these parasites, but you should remember to have your babies wear protective footwear when they are out, and don't put them on the ground or on a sandy beach without a towel or blanket to play on.

Plan—and Go!

Becoming a parent is one of the great joys of life, but having a baby doesn't mean you're grounded for life. Travel is still a good thing, but you'll need to learn how to travel smart. If you thoughtfully prepare and take the necessary precautions, vacationing far and wide with your new baby can be exciting, loads of fun, and safe.

So put your baby in your back pocket and keep exploring!

14

. . . . .

Embrace Your Tribe

Not that long ago, most people on the earth lived together in towns or villages, or on family farms. These cloistered, agrarian-based settlements were geographically minuscule, covering a landmass of no more than a handful of acres. Thus, by virtue of their proximity, the inhabitants of these towns knew their neighbors and were intimately involved in the lives of one another.

These communities were composed of individuals of all ages and were knit together by blood, religion, and shared values. Within these bustling enclaves were extended families that included grandparents, uncles, and cousins as well as mothers and fathers and their children. These were not the nuclear families that we know today but, rather, intimate human clusters where people clung to one another for survival and helped one another face the challenges that life brings.

Early globalization and the Industrial Revolution changed this old order. Large cities sprang up along the great rivers and protected ocean inlets as trade between different areas and municipalities multiplied. The small communities of yesteryear, scattered out in the hinterlands, were unable to compete with the excitement and opportunities that these larger cities offered, and thus, the small hamlets dwindled and families, who had lived together in them for generations, began to disperse.

With the advent of the twentieth century, the world changed even more. Trains, ocean liners, cars, buses, and airplanes began shuttling people around the globe safely, effortlessly, and for those who could afford it, sumptuously. Traveling was no longer a daunting and dangerous task. It had morphed into a pleasurable experience. Uprooting and taking to the road wasn't the big ordeal it had once been. It became possible for *everyone* to migrate, and human nature being what it is, that's exactly what happened. Families, looking for greater opportunities, set out to explore the unknown—and frequently, they gravitated to urban centers.

This new mobility caused the cohesive units of extended family to fragment even more. Today, in the United States, it's not uncommon to have Mom and Dad living on the East Coast while their children, in various relationships and stages of life, reside on the other side of the country or even abroad. Before, we lived atop one another in beehive villages teeming with friends and family. Now we live atop one another in tall, shiny buildings or in homes in sprawling suburbia, each with its own backyard. Our homes are protected, isolated, and somewhat dehumanized "little boxes on the hillside" next to people we don't know and with our families of origin often far, far away.

The Real Story Is More Sanguine

But this somewhat dark scenario of twenty-first-century family life is only partially true. My experience working in a highly urban, diverse community is more hopeful. I've found that family ties are still important to most young couples with new babies. I know this because when a baby is born, grandmothers and grandfathers suddenly appear out of nowhere. Aunties, uncles, and cousins magically show up too. For many people, the family unit in America is still a vibrant and living entity.

But though the heart may be fond, geographic separation represents a true challenge for family intimacy, and for those who are far removed from these close family ties, raising children can be a stressful and lonely endeavor.

One thing I encourage my young parents, those who are separated from their relatives, to consider is how they can more fully *reengage* with their extended families because family represents the first foundation that we know in life. The traditions of our youth may get buried as we leave home and move through careers, but when babies come, many couples find those quiescent embers of family tradition still smoldering. And many young parents find comfort in reacquainting themselves with these remembrances and likewise relish surrounding themselves with the people who love them the most.

Heading Home

Really reengaging with your family may require a career change or even a move across the country. This is a big deal, especially for young parents who have just had a baby, but moving back to your hometown may be the exact solution to many of the challenges new moms and dads face. I have had several young families in my practice move to where their social support is centered. In doing so, they have found that raising children is less lonely and much more doable. Having friends and your extended family surrounding you as you raise your children is immeasurably valuable.

Move Your Family to You!

There are other ways to get your extended family back into your life. Rather than moving back to their hometowns, many families in my practice have done the very opposite. Dangling delightful and impossibly cute grandchildren in front of their parents' eyes, they've enticed their parents, and other relatives as well, to move closer to them.

This is equally wonderful. Grandparents, some who are widowed or living alone, find that moving out of their empty nests to be closer to their children and grandchildren gives them a fresh boost. Let it be known that grandchildren are a blessing to grandparents.

Living Together with Your Parents

Other families have taken other creative steps. One family in my practice was living with the mother's parents for several years. Their goal was to save enough money for a down payment on a home in the grandparents' neighborhood. Judging from my observations and the reports they have given me, things have worked out quite well. The maternal grandmother is the primary caretaker when Mommy is at work, and financially, they saved a bundle. During a recent appointment with this family, I was told some happy news: by living with her parents, they were able to save enough to buy their first house in the same neighborhood as her parents.

For this family, their plan turned out to be a win-win!

Another family in my practice bought the home next door to the mother's parents' house. They then proceeded to tear down the fence that separated their two adjacent properties, and in doing so, they created one large, contiguous backyard. Their two children now have oodles of room to roam between the two homes, two places where they are welcome and dearly loved. As an aside, this family is particularly happy. When the mother brings her children in, she appears rested and wears a sweet smile, and the grandmother, who frequently comes along to her grandchildren's appointments, is also a cheery and content woman. The children are likewise thriving and happy. Something very wonderful is working in this family. Maybe it's just who they are, but I also have a hunch that their happiness has something to do with how they have structured their lives and how they synergistically help one another.

The concept of family members helping one another out applies to other family members as well. Having uncles and aunts close by is equally valuable to parents and enriching to children. To consummate these kinds of living arrangements, however, takes planning and, for some, sacrifice. But family is family, and blood still counts.

Grandparents Are a Blessing to Grandchildren

I was one of those who grew up with a paucity of grandparent input. Three of my grandparents were deceased by the time I was born, and the one grandfather I did have lived far away, so my times with him were limited. Nevertheless, I remember him well. The cousins all called him Grumpy, although he was anything but grumpy, and he lived with my aunt, my uncle, and two of my cousins. His routine was to take a daily walk in the neighborhood, and then, after coming home, he would recline in an oversized armchair and smoke a pipe.

Grumpy's pipe smoking enthralled me as a young kid. No one else in my life smoked a pipe, and I remember watching with rapt attention as he packed his pipe with tobacco and then lit it with a long wooden match. The blue smoke from his small inferno filled the room with a pleasant aroma that I still remember today. This was how my kind and laconic Swedish grandfather enjoyed himself.

In addition to pipe smoking, when we visited, he had another routine. In turn, he would sit me and each of my four siblings on his knee, hug us, give us a Nordic "peep-tucka-tuck" squeeze on the nose and murmur to us in his deep Swedish accent something I never really understood. Then he would pull out his money pouch and present to each of us a shiny silver dollar. I particularly loved the silver dollar routine, and seeing my delight, Grumpy predicted that I was destined to someday become a banker. Although he was wise and revered, he missed on that one. My banking career never quite took off, but I still have a penchant for silver dollars.

Although I never interacted with my grandfather as much as I would have liked, looking back, I see the wonderful and positive input he had in my life. I am a richer and more fulfilled man today because I knew him. Thanks to my parents, who made it a priority for us to visit Grumpy, knowing him gave me a broader perspective of life and produced in me a knowledge of my heritage, a thread that still links me back to the old country of Sweden.

The Gift of Grandparents

Grandparents around the globe play vital roles in caring for their grandchildren. This is true in the United States as well. Working moms and dads find great solace in having their own parents care for their babies, knowing that grandparents are, in most cases, totally committed to their children's children. Parents know that the quality of the care for their children could not be better than with another family member.

But babysitting your child isn't the only gift grandparents bring to the picture. Without grandparents, your children would be missing out on the blessings of elder wisdom. People learn things as they age. They look back over their lives and realize, sometimes with great regret, all the mess-ups they have made. This is normal. We learn from these mistakes, and grandparents bring this hard-earned wisdom with them when they come into the lives of their grandchildren.

But older people also bring with them stories of things that *went right* and other tales of adventure and conquest: like the investment that everyone else laughed at that turned into a giant windfall or the random trip to Greece that not only brought wonderful adventure but also led to a Grecian romance and, ultimately, a Greek wife! These are the repeated yarns that grandparents tell and that, when they do so, enrich their grandchildren immeasurably and add to the fabric that unites families.

Who's in Charge?

An important consideration for families when members of the extended family, *including grandparents*, care for their children is this: Who's in charge?

The answer to this question is easy, except in rare cases: *moms and dads are in charge*. You're the ones who maintain and set the boundaries in your home. You're the ultimate authority in your household. This is the proper order of things.

Scheduling, feedings, sleep times, and even disciplinary practices are under the direction of the child's parents. Grandmothers and grandfathers must understand this, and for the great majority of grandparents whom I know, this is not a problem.

If you do find that you are having difficulties with the way your extended family is caring for your child (perhaps they are feeding her food you prefer she not eat), stand up for yourself and share with your family caregivers your feelings and thoughts. Explain to them why you want to raise your child the way you do.

In the end, they are *your* children.

Don't Overwork the Grandparents

Most grandparents relish the opportunity to care for their grandchildren. For grandparents who care for their grandchildren on a full-time basis, however, there is a limit. Studies show that grandparents find caregiving less pleasant if the workload exceeds thirty hours per week.

These same studies have found that overutilization of grandparents has a negative effect on their health and their sense of well-being. So, moms and dads who rely on your parents to help you, be sensitive not to overburden grandparents.

Here are some facts about the role of grandparents in the lives of their grandchildren:

- Grandparents play a significant role in providing childcare around the globe, especially for single, working parents.
- Grandparents are the main childcare providers for 35 percent of families where moms work or are in school. Moms and dads have a strong preference for this arrangement.
- Few grandparents provide full-time care. Most care for the grandchildren ten hours per week or fewer.
- Moms who return to work within six months of their babies being born utilize grandparents more extensively. This is particularly true for single moms.
- Grandparents continue to have significant roles after children enter school, especially during holiday periods.
- Most grandparents enjoy caring for their grandchildren if they are not called upon to do it on a full-time basis.
- Close contact to grandparents, especially maternal grandparents, is associated with healthier child adjustment to other situations. Studies show that individuals who had

278 > 7 Secrets of the Newborn

strong ties to their grandparents as children suffered less depression as adolescents and young adults.

Seven Benefits Extended Families Enjoy

Extended family members:

1. Are role models and positive influences for children.
2. Provide children with a sense of encouragement, security, and stability.
3. Help children better understand the roots of their families.
4. Let children know that there are people outside the immediate family who love and care about them.
5. Provide advice or act as a support system for parents.
6. Help build on the sense of community for the child.
7. Provide emergency babysitting in a pinch.

Your Extended Family Might Not Be Family

While many new mommies and daddies have parents or extended family they can rely on, not everyone is so fortunate. If you have close friends, however, who can fill a family role, your child will receive some of the same benefits from their presence as they do from actual family. Best friends, whom you have known "pre-child," can suddenly become "uncles" and "aunties" to your little flock, and many show the same love and affection as your blood relatives. Embrace and nourish these relationships to the benefit of your baby.

When Leslie and I moved to Los Angeles for me to attend medical school, we found ourselves alone in a big city. We had no family in the Southern California area, and as our family grew, it became more challenging for us to travel the hundreds of miles back and forth to our families for the holidays. When we realized the truth of this situation, we began sharing Thanksgivings and many of the other holidays and weekends with our friends Leon and Susan, whom we knew before we were married. This led to a relationship that has endured for more than forty years.

Leon and Susan filled in for our extended family as we shared all the major holidays with them and their boys. We blended our families together, and as the years have passed, there has hardly been a holiday that has gone by where our friends have not been a part of the celebration. Susan and Leon love our children like they love their own, and we feel the same warmth and connection with their boys as well.

Siblings Are Part of the Fun

I tell my patients when they have their first child, "You don't have a child, you have a family!" *Your* family may currently contain only one child, but most families (80 percent) go on to have more than one. Siblings represent one of the longest relationships a person will have in his or her lifetime and are a source of great support for one another. The relationship between blood relatives runs deep, so brothers and sisters are meant to be there to help us when we are in need. This begins when we are young children and continues, in many cases, throughout life.

While some moms and dads begin parenthood knowing they want more than one child, others are skeptical about all the difficulties additional children may bring—particularly with fighting, arguments, and sibling rivalry.

But not all sibling interactions are cantankerous. Siblings have sweet times together too. They play with each other and learn from each other. Children with siblings also experience less loneliness.

The Benefits of Having a Sibling

- Siblings teach us how to navigate the world. As researchers Nina Howe and Holly Recchia put it, "The sibling relationship is a natural laboratory for young children to learn about their world."
- Sibling relationships are often emotionally charged and uninhibited, in both positive and negative ways.
- Sibling relationships are defined by intimacy. Young children end up spending a lot of time with their siblings, playing together, and getting to know each other. This opens the door for siblings to provide emotional support to one another through the years.
- Siblings play an important role in teaching one another about understanding the emotions, thoughts, intentions, and beliefs of others.
- Siblings who engage in pretend play demonstrate a greater understanding of others' emotions.
- Conflict resolution is a big part of sibling interaction because quarrels and conflict among siblings is very common. Our rough edges are polished by the words and actions of brothers or sisters in the conflict among siblings that is inevitable.
- Lessons that can be learned through siblings include sharing and comfort that we are not alone. A sibling can become a confidant to share our thoughts with and, later in life, become that other individual to help care for aging parents.

I think it is always a good idea to at least consider having more than one child. Second and third children enrich the lives of a first child. The delight and joy of having more children and watching their interactions is also not an arithmetic jump; it is an *exponential*, logarithmic leap.

Birth Spacing and Prematurity

If you decide to have more children, the amount of time you should wait before having another baby is an important consideration. Although there has been debate over the years as to what the "best time" is to have a subsequent child, research shows that having a second child born fewer than twenty-seven months after the first increases the rates of premature birth with the subsequent, second infant, particularly in younger and older mothers, or in mothers who have hypertension or who've delivered a previous preterm child.

Fully 53 *percent* of mothers who give birth to a second child within twelve months of the first (so-called Irish twins) deliver their second children prematurely. This is a big number! Women who give birth to a second child within eighteen months (in other words, those women who get pregnant within nine months after giving birth with baby number one) likewise have higher rates of prematurity. The studies show that the optimal time interval between giving birth to one child and becoming pregnant with a second child is *eighteen months or more.*

So if you want more than one child, think about spacing, but don't wait too long to have another baby. It is common knowledge that siblings separated in age from each other by several years don't have the same intimate relationships with each other—at least during their early, formative years—as siblings who are closer in age.

As siblings age, however, a closeness grows, and as adults, siblings who were separated even by many years often become fast friends and great allies.

Family Traditions, Family Holidays, and Values

Because family is important, your family's religious traditions, cultural customs, and holiday festivities help secure and orient your child's identity. People, even young people, need to be anchored to something. Exposing and sharing with your children the traditions of your family gives them a sense of belonging to a larger group and yields countless benefits.

Children also learn manners, ethics, civility, morals, discipline, self-restraint, and honor within the context of their families. Other values like honesty, thrift, responsibility, and respect for authority are likewise learned by close example. Serving the homeless at a Thanksgiving soup kitchen, bringing a meal to a grieving family, and visiting the sick in the hospital are taught in the context of both your nuclear family and your extended family. So embrace your family and the unique traditions that make your family special and let your children share the rich heritage that you know.

Children Bring the Estranged Back Together Again

For some, returning to one's family and roots will entail the re-establishment and restoration of relationships that, over the course of time and events, have become estranged. This is another secret, another of those positive happenings that babies help bring to pass. Babies not only adorn our world with light and life, they bring healing and redemption.

If you have fallen out with your family, seek ways to repair and mend your relationship with them. If for no other reason, do this for your sake of your child. Everyone benefits when families are brought back together again.

Embracing Your Tribe

While society has moved far from those distant times when it was assumed that the members of the clan would support one another when babies were born, the moms and dads of today should do their best to avoid going it alone. Open (and in some cases reopen) your heart to your family and sense and see the love that will surround your baby.

It's a wonderful thing.

Remember too that family isn't an option—it is an imperative. It's the first community your child will ever know.

Carl Jung put it this way: "The little world of childhood with its familiar surroundings is a model of the greater world. The more intensively the family has stamped its character upon the child, the more [the child] will tend to feel and see its earlier miniature world again in the bigger world of adult life."

15

. . . . .

Relax, Retreat, and Reenergize

Secret #7: We All Need Rest, Especially New Mothers and Fathers

Joseph Lieberman, the former U.S. senator from Connecticut, was one of the busiest individuals in the nation during his tenure in government service. But despite the frenetic schedule that being a senator entails, he nevertheless made a practice of extracting himself from the chaos of government service at sunset every Friday evening so he could take a Sabbath rest. It was a feat that he had to strategically plan for and intentionally work toward throughout his week, but he did it, and he did it faithfully—to the astonishment of many.

During Lieberman's years in Washington, D.C., reporters and constituents, wondering about his commitment to this weekend routine, frequently asked him, "Mr. Lieberman, how can you stop all your work as a senator to observe the Sabbath?" His answer was instructive: "How can I do all my work as a senator if I *do not stop* and observe the Sabbath?" Putting down his cell phone, turning his computer off, and stepping away from the fray of political life was exactly what the senator needed to successfully fulfill the responsibilities he daily shouldered. In his book *The Gift of Rest*, Lieberman explained that taking a Sabbath rest was more than just a curious tradition; for him, it was *restorative*.

If an astute, accomplished, and insanely busy senator needs downtime from his responsibilities, maybe there's a lesson here for parents of young children as well. Perhaps it's a bit of a stretch to compare being a parent of a young child to being a United States senator, but there are parallels. Both jobs impact concretely the lives of others, entail an unrelenting full-time schedule of tasks, and require your physical presence. And finally, both jobs require responding to demanding constituents! Senators' phones ring incessantly between votes and meetings. Mothers and fathers have babies in need of something at all hours, every day of the week.

So the lesson Senator Lieberman teaches is this: taking a break and getting away from the intensity of it all are necessary, no matter how tough you think you are.

> *In the tempestuous ocean of time and toil there are islands of stillness where man may enter a harbor and reclaim his dignity. The island is the seventh day, the Sabbath, a day of detachment from things, instruments, and practical affairs, as well as of attachment to the spirit.*
>
> —ABRAHAM JOSHUA HESCHEL, *THE SABBATH*

Pace Yourself

I don't necessarily consider myself much of a runner, but I have managed to complete a handful of marathons over the past several years. I don't run, however, quite like the other young bucks who go zipping by me. Instead, I trudge. Pity is the emotion I induce in most people who see me making my way down the road. No one seeing me is overly impressed, and nobody has ever broken through the crowd to shake my hand.

But that's okay, because I know who I am. I am a sixty-plus-year-old pediatrician. I know my limits, and thus, I get through the marathon by running what the pros call *intervals*. This is a dressed-up, fancy way of saying that *I rest a lot* during the journey. And if the truth be spoken, this is the *only* way that I make it to the finish line.

Some years ago, I decided to endeavor to live my life with a simple philosophy: if it's good enough for God, it's good enough for me too. With this as my underlying ethos, I constructed a biblical model to structure my marathon run. Genesis, the first book of the Torah, says that God spent six days creating the heavens and earth and then, on the seventh day, *he rested*. With this as a template, I've developed what I call the *biblical creation marathon model* for running. It goes like this: I run for six minutes, and then I rest by taking a one-minute walk. It's a simple scheme.

While taking this one-minute rest, I doff my cap, mop my brow, and catch my breath. And during these mini-breaks, mini-miracles occur. My mind clears, and I get perspective. I look up to see the sky and behold the clouds. I hear barking dogs, songbirds high above me in the trees, and the shouts of encouragement from the crowd that lines each side of the road. In addition, this short respite allows me an opportunity to take in the bigger picture of all the things that are going on around me, which is otherwise impossible to do while running.

This brief break also grants me just enough time to slurp down a splash of Gatorade and get refreshed. So when sixty seconds have elapsed and it's time to start running again, I'm ready (and willing) to get moving.

That's my pattern. Six on, one off. Time and time again, hour after hour.

Finally, after five hours of plodding, twenty-six long miles have peeled away, and miraculously, I'm done!

Am I exhausted?

Absolutely! But finishing the run brings me such a sense of accomplishment that this exhaustion feels good. Every marathon runner will tell you that. For me, as I receive accolades from family and friends, I quietly know in my heart that my "Sabbath" breaks made the difference.

Moms and Dads Need Sleep

Raising children is no different from running a marathon. It's not a sprint; it's a long journey that requires a strategy. Getting enough rest should be part of the plan, but for most of my patients' families, things usually start out a bit rocky, and restorative rest is hard to come by.

At the one-month well-child visit to my office, after I have gone through the questions about their babies with the new parents, I like to turn to them and ask them how *they* are doing. Their response is almost invariably the same: *"We're beat!"*

New parents are easy to spot. They're the ones who walk around bleary-eyed and dazed, refugees from the front. They're utterly pooped! One of the most compelling needs for moms and dads in the first months of life with baby—and the thing that they all lack—is sleep.

According to sleep specialists, adults need between seven and nine hours of sleep a day to be healthy. Those who repeatedly fail to meet this need lack mental sharpness and accrue a "sleep debt." For new parents, that debt calculates out to be nearly 350 hours during the first year.

Sleep specialist William Dement, M.D., reports that parents lose around two hours of sleep a day during the first five months after a child is born. After this, the sleep loss goes down to approximately one hour per day until their child is two years of age. But for the first few months, parents are constantly exhausted. Breastfeeding moms bear the brunt of this sleep deficit. As one mother said to me, "I was sleepwalking for the first two months of my child's life." She isn't alone.

Fortunately, things usually start getting better by three to four months. By this age, most infants are sleeping longer stretches at night, and moms have adjusted their sleep schedules to match the schedules of their children.

Interestingly, when things calm down sleep-wise, some mothers, despite the fatigue that they felt during those first months, look back nostalgically and miss the tender late-night and early-morning bonding moments they had with their babies. Most moms, however, are just happy to have that stage of infancy over!

But there are ways to help moms and dads get more sleep and to help get your baby to sleep longer throughout the night. Here are some ideas that will assist you in recapturing some of those 350 hours of sleep that parents lose during the first year of a baby's life:

- **Make your sleeping arrangement comfortable.** Have a good mattress and keep the room at a comfortable temperature.
- **Allow light into your baby's room during the day, but at night, make baby's sleep environment as dark as possible.** This helps your baby sleep better. If your baby is sleeping longer, you reap a tangible reward.
- **Gently guide your baby into a schedule that coincides with yours.** Even in the newborn stage, you can begin scheduling feeding, playing, bathing, and sleeping.
- **Take a nap!** Resist the temptation to clean up and do chores when your baby is napping. Sleep when your baby sleeps. To heck with trying to maintain a perfect house

during this time. There is nothing wrong with living like a bohemian for a couple of months, especially if the trade-off is some more sleep. Researchers say that even a twenty-minute nap can refresh, and a forty-five-minute nap can increase your alertness for another six hours. For working moms, take a nap during your lunch hour.

- **Enlist others to watch your baby while you take a nap.** Now is the time to cash in on all the favors people owe you. Trusted friends and family can make all the difference in the world during these times.
- **Don't look at the clock while you are in bed.** Fixation on the clock only induces anxiety.
- **Avoid caffeine, nicotine, and alcohol for six hours before bedtime.** Both caffeine and nicotine are stimulants, and although alcohol is a depressant, it paradoxically disrupts sleep patterns by causing more wakefulness later in the night.
- **Avoid exercising three hours before bedtime.** Exercise releases energizing endorphins that enhance your sense of well-being, but they also hype you up and cause your brain to spin. Get your exercise in the morning to help promote restful sleep at night.
- **Sleep with your baby in your room.** When baby wakes up at night, it helps to have him readily accessible to feed. This avoids those stumbling treks to the nursery in the middle of the night. After you are done feeding, however, it's important that you put your baby back into his bassinet on his back. Remember too that it is imperative that a nursing mother *not fall asleep* with her baby in bed or in a lounge chair. The American Academy of Pediatrics recommends that parents sleep in the same room with their babies until the babies are six months of age.

- **Pre-fill a couple of bottles before bedtime and put them nearby** for those middle-of-the-night feedings. If you are formula feeding your baby, freshly mixed formula, which you prepare before your bedtime, will keep and be fine for your baby when he awakes during the night. (Likewise, freshly pumped breast milk will keep for this relatively short period and can be given by Dad to help Mommy get a few extra winks of rest.)

- **Avoid screen time before sleeping.** Computers, video screens, televisions, and even your beloved cell phone emit 470 nm of light waves. This wavelength looks like blue light to the brain and has a stimulatory effect by causing a decrease in melatonin secretion. If you want to read before bedtime, find a book.

- **Room temperature matters.** People fall asleep better with cooler room temperatures. Sixty-five degrees Fahrenheit is a good, round number to shoot for. This is okay for baby too, provided he is adequately dressed.

SURPRISE: Sleep Helps with Pregnancy Weight Loss

Q: Can getting more sleep actually help me lose pregnancy pounds?
A: Yes! While a good night of sleep is necessary to feel refreshed and energized, it can also help you lose any extra weight you might be carrying from your pregnancy:

- Moms who get more than five hours of sleep per night lose their pregnancy weight more quickly than those who do not.
- Women who do not get enough sleep after delivery retain more than eleven pounds of pregnancy weight at one year postpartum.

Sleeplessness and Babies Bring New Stresses to Marriage

Check out the baby blogs and parenting magazines and you will notice that almost every issue has at least one story of the challenges and stresses that babies bring to a marital relationship. In a *Wall Street Journal* article, writer Andrea Peterson put it this way: "A couple's satisfaction with their marriage takes a nosedive after the first child is born. Sleepless nights and fights over whose turn it is to change diapers can leach the fun out of a relationship." Studies dating back to the 1950s show that most marriages experience a crisis in the transitional months after babies come, but it doesn't take a study to know that this is true. It only takes a baby.

The most precious relationship in life, the one that young parents should do all they can do to preserve, is marriage. A healthy and thriving marriage is also critical for the growth, development, and happiness of your child. You may *do all the right things* for your child, like fully vaccinate her, feed her only the best organic and nutritious foods, limit her television time, and set clear bedtime hours, but if your marriage dies, much of the good that you have done for your child will come to naught.

When babies are born, your life is rocked, and all that you do begins to revolve around a different center. These changes are unavoidable, and for the most part, they are good, but inevitably, they will affect your marriage to the point that some mothers even admit to "hating" their spouses. *Hate* is a strong word. Those new moms who confess to these feelings say they find themselves snapping at their partners for everything and find that they become overly judgmental and irritated by silly things that never bothered them before. Niceties like *thank you* and *please* get dropped from their conversations.

One reflective mother later asked herself, "Why was my husband so annoying? Here was the person I loved, with whom I had just pulled off the miracle of creating a life and . . . I wanted to kill him." Women report a general negative sense about their marriages early on, usually within the first six months after delivery. Men say that they can sense negativity even earlier.

Cultivating Your Marriage by Taking a "Parental Sabbath" . . . Without Baby

Fully two-thirds of couples see the quality of their relationship drop within three years after their first child, but having your marriage sour after a baby comes *should not* be a given. To keep marriage a happy and vibrant relationship, it must be intentionally nourished and cultivated.

A major component of this marriage dissatisfaction is due to sleep deprivation and the new roles that new parents must assume. Stress in a marriage is completely understandable when people are both overwhelmed and sleep deprived. There's too much to do and too little time in which to do it and therefore relationships can go sideways and get wonky very quickly. Let's face it: it's hard to connect with your spouse when there's a baby screaming in the background.

So getting a break from the war zone helps ward off a lot of the negative feelings partners feel toward each other. Hence, it's important to strategically schedule times moms and dads can spend time together . . . *without* baby.

The first step is to *make a plan*. As the saying goes, "Those who fail to plan, plan to fail." So from time to time, parents need to look ahead on the calendar and set some time away. Stepping away from the task of parenting and enjoying time together alone or with friends, *without the minute-by-minute demands of caring for a child*, is refreshing.

So schedule a date. Go to dinner. Enjoy a movie. Call friends and have a meal together. Early on, these will be very short breaks—most will be a couple of hours at the max—because your baby needs you, but by the end of the first year, things get better. Believe it or not, you'll be able to take short overnight, weekend vacations without your child. So don't despair—there's hope coming.

Finally, micro-moments, like taking a few minutes to walk around the block or running down to the ice cream shop for a soda—alone, without your baby—can provide the extra boost in your day that will help you survive.

I consider this all part of good parenting practices. Those who pace themselves and make taking a "parental Sabbath" a part of their routines will be rewarded, rejuvenated, and, when the rest is over, ready to get back into the parenting game.

Forgetting Who You Are!

Perhaps I'm stretching things too far, but if you're lucky, you might, during one of these rare minutes away, even forget that you are a parent! Possibly, you'll have a conversation with friends that goes beyond diapers and breastfeeding. Maybe the movie you see will transport you to a different planet and drop you off. Or perhaps that two-hour afternoon nap will come with some sweet dreams.

Don't count on forgetting your responsibilities for too long, however. Babies have a way of gnawing away at your brain, and ultimately, they even conquer your unconscious mind. They may not be in your immediate presence, but your every thought is directed toward them.

I know this seems counter to all that I have been espousing in this book, but I really hope it happens to you. And don't feel guilty if it does! That said, I assure you, if your mind does wander, you won't be able to revel in this state of denial for long. Your parental role will come crashing back on your head the second you walk through your front door. Babies specialize in keeping parents focused and in the moment.

How to Find the Right Babysitter

If you don't have close family or friends who can watch your baby for you while you spend some alone time with your spouse, you may be able to find a babysitter. Here are some pointers on getting the right one:

- **Personal recommendations** are the best source of reliable and excellent babysitters.
- **Organizations like churches and synagogues you attend and trust** can be a great place to find a willing babysitter.
- **Childcare agencies have lists of excellent people,** but you will be charged a fee to access them.
- **Interview your prospective babysitter, get references, and call these references.** Make sure the babysitter you hire is current in CPR and first-aid skills. When she comes to interview, is she on time? Finally, how well did she interact with your child, and did your child respond well to her?

Laughing Through the Fight

Another important facet of pacing during parenthood is humor. It's medicinal to laugh, to laugh hard, and to laugh long. I am fortunately married to a woman who has managed to keep me laughing on a daily basis. Leslie's timing is second to none, and everyone who knows her will attest that her giggly wit is legendary. She's funny, and we leverage her humor—and occasionally (rarely) even mine—to make each day a bit sweeter. One mommy blogger recommended that couples should "take ten to fifteen minutes every day to laugh." I can't add anything to that good advice.

Eight Ideas for Young Parents

1. Look for free events listed in your local newspaper to see if there is anything that sounds interesting and fun for the both of you . . . then just go!
2. Visit your local art museum.
3. Exercise together. If you've never done it before, now may be a good time to start. Burn some calories and spend some time together. Couples who get fit together stay together.
4. Pick your own produce. While this one does cost a few bucks, you're actually paying for the produce you take home. Look for a local farm or orchard where you can pick your own strawberries, apples, oranges, and more.
5. Volunteer together at your favorite local charity. Feel good, do good, help out, and spend some entirely cost-free quality time together while simultaneously making the world a better place.
6. Go for coffee. It's amazing how terrific a simple, quiet cup of coffee for two is after many days in the parenting trenches. Same applies to a bagel, a doughnut, or an ice cream.
7. Take a walk together in your neighborhood or a nearby park.
8. Swap quiet time. Take your kiddo to a friend's so you can have a few hours at your own home, then take your friend's baby so she can do the same.

A Sabbath Rest

When I was a child, Americans lived under the so-called blue laws. These were laws that hearkened back to our Puritan roots and strictly forbid businesses to be open on Sundays. For those rare businesses that *were* allowed to be open on Sundays, like pharmacies and restaurants, the blue laws restricted their hours of operation and even what products they were allowed to sell. In many states, for example, alcoholic beverages could not be sold on Sundays. Other states forbade the selling of automobiles.

As a child, I didn't understand the origins of these laws, but I knew that Sunday was a different day. My parents called Sunday the Lord's Day, not only for our family but for the entire community.

I remember Sundays as being peaceful days. No one mowed their lawns or washed their cars. Traffic was minimal, and the vehicles that were on the road seemed to go slower. No one seemed to be in a hurry. The only equivalent I can think of today is Christmas morning. The quietude that prevails in our cities and towns on Christmas morning was exactly how Sundays felt *every week*.

Sunday was America's Sabbath Day. People went to church and then came home to a large midday family meal. They took naps, read books, went on walks, reflected, and rejuvenated. Quiet Sundays were simply part of the culture of the community. People inherently understood the value and the importance of resting. In fact, it was the law!

Senator Lieberman put it this way in his final chapter of his book: "We live in a culture of hard work where people are desperately in need of rest, not just rest to recharge our batteries so we can work harder, but to recharge our souls so we can live better. For me, the answer to that need has been the Sabbath. It has anchored my life, revived my body, and restored my soul."

Apply the Blue Laws to Your Baby Too

It would be wonderful if there were blue laws that governed our babies. These innocent yet all-consuming little rascals don't understand, nor do they seem to care, that their parents are at the tattered edges of sanity when they start screaming at two o'clock in the morning. This is the nature of new babies, and you must deal with these interruptions to meet the needs of your child. But equally important is finding times to withdraw from the fray. Rest is a foundational stone in the art of parenting, and it should be factored into the equation if parents plan on winning the game.

So protect your sanity and reinforce your marriage by giving yourself a parental "Sabbath"—a self-proclaimed day (or weekend) of rest—and make it a habit. Schedule rests frequently into your busy lives; take a break and you will be rewarded. Find yourselves an excellent babysitter whom you can trust. Treat her well and pay her well, and she'll come back.

And while you are at it, put down your cell phone and close up your laptop too.

Epilogue

· · · · ·

The Blessing of Children

Bonus Secret: Babies Are Even More Fun Than You Can Imagine—It's All Worth It

This is a pro-child book. I've written it in an attempt to dazzle my readers with *life:* its mysterious wonder, its miraculous nature, and the blessing that a new life brings to parents and the world.

Babies really are the best!

But is it easy to be a parent? *No!*

Will you have enough money in your pocket to pay for everything? *No!*

Will it be total chaos in your house? *Yes!*

Should you wait until you have it all together to have a baby? *No!* (You'll never really have it all together anyway—and when the baby comes, he'll surely mess up any pretense that you *thought* was "together.")

So is it still worth it . . . knowing in advance what's about to happen to your "perfect" life?

Absolutely yes!

Why? *Because babies are wonderful!*

They're our future, and they bring hope.

And even if you have thought that having a baby is impossible, it's not.

It's completely doable and an exciting venture for young couples who have the courage, the resolve, and the pluck to step out in faith.

As one mother put it, "It's the hardest job you will ever love."

We're All Naive

Cheerleading aside, I want my readers to also know that I'm not for blindly doing *anything*, much less bringing a child into this world willy-nilly. That's called making bad choices and foolishness, and this is never a good tactic to live by *or* espouse. But a "calculated risk," as General George Patton once said, "is quite different from being rash."

Being rash leads to problems, but being *naive* and taking what Patton would call "a calculated risk" is a different thing. Everyone is naive when they venture into unknown territory, but diving in and bumping up against reality is how we grow, how we learn, and how we mature beyond naiveté.

Consider, for a Moment, a World with No Children

In the Japanese village of Hara-izumi, bears, deer, and wild boar roam the streets where children once played. It's just one of many towns and villages across the island nation that have been hollowed out as Japan's population dwindles.

The decline in the Japanese population is a phenomenon that is widely known and well documented. A recent front-page story in the *Los Angeles Times* painted a sad picture of temples abandoned and factories shuttered. Every year, the country closes five hundred schools for lack of students, and transportation officials now deliberate over which rural roads they plan to maintain and which roads they will allow to revert to nature.

At its peak in 2010, Japan's population reached 128 million people, but with this generation's birth decline, they are losing 1 million people each year. Demographic experts predict that the nation's population will drop by 40 million by 2060, leaving Japan with a population of 88 million individuals. This is an unprecedented *30 percent decline* in one generation.

Fewer citizens is only half of the demographic concerns for Japan. An even more ominous challenge is Japan's aging population. By the middle of this century, 40 percent of people living in Japan will be over sixty-five years of age. The economic ramifications of a population bubble of septuagenarians and octogenarians is vast and far-reaching. Retirees and partial-working older people tend to be neither income producers nor consumers. Elderly people don't purchase much in the way of houses, cars, or other goods, and therefore, domestic markets dry up.

The Chinese Have the Same Conundrum

Farther south and to the west, on the Asian continent, lies China. For thirty-five years, the People's Republic of China vigorously enforced a one-child policy to curb what it considered an overabundance of people. This policy was reversed in January 2015 after officials realized that their nation was soon to face a stark reality. China, the home of a seemingly never-ending supply of workers, is heading toward a serious mid-twenty-first-century manpower shortage that will number in the tens of millions of people.

The slow churn and unforgiving demographic curve the Chinese forgot to factor into their future is about to catch up with them and bitterly bite them as they limp into a child-barren future.

But it doesn't stop there. A derivative of China's one-child policy and an unforeseen secondary consequence of the country's newfound prosperity is a dearth of marriage. Despite the reversal of the one-child policy, Chinese young people aren't jumping into beds and making babies. They are doing the very opposite. Those who are getting married are putting it off longer than ever, and many young Chinese aren't taking the step at all. Last year, only 12 million couples, in a nation of 1.4 billion people, registered to marry, fewer than the year before, which was also fewer than the year before that.

And with fewer marriages come fewer children.

What was once denied to them by their government, the young people of China are now voluntarily opting to continue—namely, delaying both marriage and having children. One of the reasons for this societal shift has been the prosperity that China is enjoying. Prosperity in a nation—and this is true around the world—often comes with a reduction in its fertility rate. But in China specifically, this trend also represents *demographic inertia*, a spillover of their government's long-enforced, one-child policy.

The net result for the People's Republic of China will be exactly what it has become in Japan over the past decade: a dearth of people.

My wife and I were recently in Beijing. It is a gigantic, bustling city filled with people. Construction cranes dot the smoggy skies on every horizon. It's hard for people visiting there today to imagine anything but a bright economic future. But demography doesn't lie. Despite the building boom that visitors see throughout the city, the immediate future for Beijing, and China, in general, is a dwindling population and economic challenge.

Sadly, nations where the population is in decline are nations that are dying a slow death.

American Demographics

One doesn't need to travel to Asia to see what is happening demographically all around the world. Europe, South America, and even the United States are all experiencing a similar downturn in fertility.

The United States Census Bureau recently reported that the American population grew only 0.7 percent from July 1, 2015 to July 1, 2016. This was the lowest growth in the U.S. population since the Great Depression, and it is predicted to continue. Demographers now predict that people older than sixty-five years of age will outnumber children in the U.S. by 2025. Already, the American workforce, those individuals between twenty-five years of age and fifty-four years of age, is shrinking.

California's fertility rate is now at its lowest level ever recorded. Eight of our fifty states are losing population due both to emigration out and depressed fertility rates within. Like Japan, the population of the United States, without robust immigration, would soon be in decline.

SURPRISE: Every woman you have ever met—your mom, your aunts, your cousins, and all of your girlfriends—must have 2.1 children in their lifetimes to maintain a population from slipping. Currently, many Western nations, including the United States, are falling below this replacement number.

Why Bring Up Demography?

Why should the challenges of world demography be included in a pro-child book, and why am I concerned? Allow me to share some thoughts.

Cultures and societies are amalgamations of small communities, families, and, in their most atomic form, individuals. A culture and the norms of that culture are ultimately a reflection of what large numbers of people, living in a shared geographic area and governed by a set of unifying laws and leaders, believe about life, liberty, and the pursuit of happiness. The "culture" of a nation mirrors what individuals and families within that society think, how they live, and what they value at any given *time* within that society.

One clear truth about societies and cultures is they're never static; they are constantly evolving, and cultural change is never ending. We see this in history. The early Roman society was vastly different from the Rome that fell to the barbarians. Things that were important to one generation lose their value in successive generations.

The tussle for popular opinion is a dynamic, daily undercurrent in every society. We all know this on a micro-basis because we see how architecture, hairstyles, and décor change within a few years. We look at pictures of our parents, laugh at their "funny" glasses, and wonder aloud how anyone could have found their styles to be attractive.

Cultural changes also occur on the macro level, and discernable themes guide societies. Attitudes about life and allegiances change over time.

And this is my concern.

In today's culture, a prevailing mind-set that I am observing in my community and that has become a reality in vast swaths of our world is this: getting married and raising children is no longer a primary goal or a pursued desire for young couples. What was once a societal given has now become an option. Young couples are procrastinating the jump into the family way because our culture is telling them that there are other more important things to pursue.

Exotic international travels, professional careers, and home purchases have replaced children as more immediate and important goals. In a nutshell, having kids can wait. More people than ever before are telling our young people not to rush into having children than are encouraging them to start raising a family.

That stated, I also know that this desire to have a family for young couples isn't dead. Procreation is a yearning deeply embedded in our DNA, and despite our current culture's relegation of having babies to the back burner, it hasn't gone away.

Nevertheless, the quiescence that surrounds starting a family and having babies concerns me. It bothers me because I have seen firsthand the blessings and delights that children bring, not only to my own family but to the thousands of families I have had the privilege to serve as a pediatrician as well. I also know that cultures that have given up on having children have given up on their futures. Societies that don't value children and that don't make it possible for their young people to have children *aren't thinking right*. In the end, they will pay a heavy price for their blindness. I don't want this to happen to America.

Furthermore, if there are not children, huge segments of our economy will become obsolete. There certainly won't be any need for schools, or teachers, or minivans, or baby food companies, or summer camps, or, for that matter, ob-gyns and even pediatricians.

In a word, a world without children is *intolerable*. It's a colorless and sad world. And this is what I am fighting against!

The Far-Fetched Dream

I see some of the signs of America's demographic slide toward childlessness on a daily basis. We can't allow this to happen. This is one of the reasons I've written this book. I'm writing to encourage the young people in our society, those who feel like the dream of having a baby is tumbling out of their reach or those who haven't given it recent thought not to give up their dream. I hope to stir passions, fan into flame those dormant dreams and tell these young people that having children is still a worthy goal and that raising a family is a good thing.

Seven Secrets of the Newborn That Will Help You Decide:

Secret #1: You Are About to Fall Desperately in Love

The love that you will have for your baby is devastatingly wonderful. Even before you behold your baby and fold her into your arms, the experience for a woman to carry a child in her womb and give birth is an incredible human experience. It will leave you in ineffable awe. Yes, it's true that all the people on this earth were at one time conceived, gestated, and delivered by a mother. It happens every day. *But when it happens to you, you will be forever changed.* I'll put money on that.

Secret #2: For the First Month, Baby Leads the Way—No Schedules, No Programs, Just Baby

The first month of your baby's life is a marvel and it will zoom by. You don't need a lot of stuff during baby's first month. When you bring your baby home, there isn't too much more you need to bring through your front door other than lots of love. The first month is the time to get to know your baby. It is a huge transition period for both you and your child. I'll be honest, it's a tough month and a lot happens. Parents generally come through it exhausted, but know there is some rest and some sweet smiles coming. Don't allow yourself to fret about rigid schedules or plans. Let baby lead the way.

Secret #3: During the First Month, Your Newborn Doesn't Need Toys, Clothes, a Stroller, or Even a Crib—All Your New Baby Needs Is You!

Having a child doesn't mean that you need to go out and buy a lot of things, especially for the first month. So sit back, start fresh, live "off the grid" and avoid running out and buying all the stuff. Take this time to enjoy each day and *keep it simple*—at least for the first month.

And if you can, do your best, within the context of your lives, to have your own *cuarentena*. Lie low away from the daily grind for one month. It's a good way to begin your lifelong adventure as a parent. What your baby needs more than anything is love. Handcraft your baby and let her know, beyond anything, that you love her and she is protected.

If you are like everyone else I know, there are demands of work and life that await you, but babies aren't forever. They grow up fast.

Secret #4: Solid and Healthy Families Don't Happen by Chance—They Are Created with Deliberation

Foundations are important to a baby's health. Build your family strong by forming a robust foundation. That foundation begins with your faith. Your faith and what you believe about life take on a new significance after a baby is born. For Leslie and me, this was one of the best decisions of our lives.

In building your family's foundation, get your baby into a healthy schedule: feed her good food, get her immunized, and take her outside into the world to discover where she landed. Keep her scrubbed, but let her get dirty too. I'm not contradicting myself. Scientists have found that "outside" kids, those children who spend long hours playing in the park, have fewer allergies, less asthma, and a stronger immune system than those who spend most of their time indoors.

Secret #5: Moms and Dads Are *Equally* Important When Raising a Baby

Marriage is another essential foundation when you have children. A two-parent team provides the basis for a secure family. Stable families, not "fragile" families, offer a strength from which your children can draw. Make this the first step in your family planning.

Take the journey of parenthood hand in hand with your spouse and appreciate how different you both are when it comes to child raising. Mothers and fathers play different roles as parents and both are important in raising a happy and well-rounded child.

Remember too that babies are a blessing to your entire family, so introduce them to the whole clan. After your little man or lady gets their first round of immunizations, don't be afraid to pop on a plane, a boat, or a train and get visiting.

Secret #6: No Screens for the First Year of Your Child's Life

During the first year of your baby's life, resist the allure of screen time. When your daughter or son starts watching a screen . . . even when they are tiny babies . . . they are transformed from active learners to passive watchers. So keep the television and smartphones and tablets away from their little eyes.

Secret #7: We All Need Rest, Especially New Mothers and Fathers

Finally, throughout this remarkable and busy year, schedule time to *rest*. This is not an esoteric idea I came up with. It started at the beginning of time. At the climax of creation, God himself took a moment to rest. So follow God's lead: relax, retreat, and reenergize. It's the only way to make it through the marathon which is child raising.

Bonus Secret: Babies Are Even More Fun Than You Can Imagine—It's All Worth It

I've always been a "bridge person." The third of five children, I learned early how to relate to people who are older and those who are younger than myself. Raised in a rural community but now living in a big city, I know how to enjoy either locality with complete comfort. I have also traveled to many parts of the world rendering medical care to some of the sickest and the poorest people on this planet. Through these experiences, I have come to a deeper appreciation of the shared humanity of all people, but through my travels, I have also acted as a bridge, transferring resources from the United States to many developing nations in both Africa and Central America.

Finally, I'm now old enough to act as another kind of bridge. I've become a bridge between two different generations. And it's in this role that I have written this book.

Much of what this book contains are thoughts and ideas that were considered the norm not so long ago. Put it this way: *Nothing I have written in this book would surprise your grandparents.* They get it.

"Of course," they would say, smiling. "People insanely love their children."

"Why indeed," they would laugh. "Your family is important!"

And with open-mouthed puzzlement, they would agree that your children need you to love and care for them.

And then they would stand and ask in unison, *"Isn't this just common sense?"*

And that's my goal! I am trying to bring some of that good old-fashioned common sense about having kids back into focus. Why? Because having a baby is one of the best things that can happen to two human beings and I don't want our world's young adults to miss out.

Some of your grandparents are here with you today. Ask them if they agree. Some of your grandparents have departed this world and now constitute part of that great cloud of witnesses. Look up and ask them the same question.

Their answer, and the answer of the One who created us all, will come not in a thunderclap but in a quiet and soft whisper.

Listen carefully, with your heart open, and you will hear it.

For Further Reading

Biss, Eula. *On Immunity: An Inoculation*. Minneapolis: Graywolf Press, 2014.

Dudek, Ronald W., Ph.D. *High-Yield Embryology*. Baltimore: Lippincott Williams & Wilkins, 1996.

Eagleman, David. *The Brain: The Story of You*. New York: Pantheon, 2015.

Eliot, Lise, Ph.D. *What's Going on in There?* New York: Bantam Books, 1999.

Finlay, B. Brett, Ph.D., and Marie-Claire Arrieta, Ph.D. *Let Them Eat Dirt*. Chapel Hill, NC: Algonquin Books, 2016.

Fraiberg, Selma. *Every Child's Birthright: In Defense of Mothering*. New York: Basic Books, 1977.

Gilligan, Carol. *In a Different Voice*. Boston: Harvard University Press, 1982.

Gopnik, Alison, Ph.D., Andrew Meltzoff, Ph.D., and Patricia Kuhl, Ph.D. *The Scientist in the Crib*. New York: William Morrow, 1999.

Greene, Alan, M.D. *Feeding Baby Green*. San Francisco: Wiley, 2009.

Heschel, Rabbi Abraham Joshua. *The Wisdom of Heschel*. 1975.

Huffington, Arianna. *The Sleep Revolution*. New York: Harmony Books, 2016.

Jana, Laura, M.D., and Jennifer Shu, M.D. *Food Fights*. 2nd ed. American Academy of Pediatrics, 2012.

Karen, Robert, Ph.D. *Becoming Attached*. New York: Warner Books, 1994.

Karp, Harvey, M.D. *The Happiest Baby on the Block*. 2nd ed. New York: Bantam, 2015.

Kersting, Thomas. *Disconnected*. 2016.

Kick, Russ, ed. *Quotes That Will Change Your Life*. Newburyport, MA: Conari Press, 2017.

Komisar, Erica, LCSW. *Being There*. New York: TarcherPerigee, 2017.

Last, Jonathan V. *What to Expect When No One's Expecting*. New York: Encounter Books, 2013.

Lieberman, Senator Joe. *The Gift of Rest*. New York: Simon & Schuster, 2011.

McRaven, Admiral William H. *Make Your Bed*. New York: Grand Central, 2017.

Medina, John. *Brain Rules for Baby*. 2nd ed. Seattle, WA: Pear Press, 2014.

Meek, Joan Younger, M.D. *New Mother's Guide to Breastfeeding*. American Academy of Pediatrics, 2011.

Miller, Lisa, Ph.D. *The Spiritual Child*. New York: St. Martin's Press, 2015.

Murkoff, Heidi, with Sharon Mazel. *What to Expect the First Year*. New York: Workman, 2014.

Murkoff, Heidi, and Sharon Mazel. *What to Expect When You're Expecting*. 5th ed. New York: Workman, 2016.

Nilsson, Lennart, and Lars Hamberger. *A Child Is Born*. 4th ed. New York: Delacorte Press, 2003.

Patel, Aniruddh D., Ph.D. *Music and the Brain*. The Great Courses, audiobook. The Teaching Company, LLC, 2015.

Peterson, Jordan B., Ph.D. *12 Rules for Life*. Canada: Random House Canada, 2018.

Port, David, John Ralston, and Brian M. Ralston, M.D. *Caveman's Guide to Baby's First Year*. New York: Sterling, 2008.

Schlessinger, Laura, Ph.D. *In Praise of Stay-at-Home Moms*. New York: HarperCollins, 2009.

Shelov, Steven P., M.D., ed. *Your Baby's First Year*. 4th ed. American Academy of Pediatrics, 2015.

Shonkoff, Jack, and Deborah Phillips, eds. *From Neurons to Neighborhoods*. National Academies Press, 2000.

Shulevitz, Judith. *The Sabbath World*. New York: Random House, 2010.

Siegel, Daniel J., M.D., and Tina Payne Bryson, Ph.D. *The Whole-Brain Child*. New York: Delacorte Press, 2011.

Spangler, Amy, R.N., M.N. *Breastfeeding: Keep It Simple*. 3rd ed., revised. 2012.

Spock, Benjamin, M.D. *Dr. Spock's Baby and Child Care*. 9th ed. New York: Pocket Books, 2011.

Stamm, Jill, Ph.D. *Boosting Brain Power.* Lewisville, NC: Gryphon House, 2016.

Stamm, Jill, Ph.D., with Paula Spencer. *Bright from the Start.* New York: Gotham Books, 2007.

Waldburger, Jennifer, LCSW, and Jill Spivack, LCSW. *The Sleepeasy Solution.* Deerfield Beach, FL: Health Communications, Inc., 2007.

Zachry, Anne H., Ph.D. *Retro Baby.* American Academy of Pediatrics, 2014.

Acknowledgments

Writing a book, I have found, is really a group effort. This was certainly true for *7 Secrets of the Newborn*. From the very start, this book has been shepherded along by many, but it was my St. Martin's editor, Nichole Argyres, who was the one who initiated the process by suggesting that I consider writing a book about children. Nichole was the true provocateur of this project, and I will forever thank her for getting it rolling and believing that maybe there was a book "inside of me" somewhere.

From there, I engaged the services of Sally Collings, an experienced writer who became the individual who organized me and encouraged me on a daily basis throughout this journey. Sally prodded me to think deeper, and then helped shape my thoughts when I did. She aided me in putting these thoughts on paper and then cleaned up my messy grammar after I did. In essence, Sally made me look and sound better than I really do, and as I confessed to her more than once, *she protected me from myself*. Thank you, Sally, for your essential role in bringing this book to fruition.

And then there were the many others who were there quietly sparking ideas in my head, sometimes without even knowing that

I was leaning on them for insight. Included in this group are my Pacific Ocean Pediatric colleagues: Leian Chen, M.D., Noel Salyer, M.D., Kelly Sidhpura, M.D., and my nurses and office staff who endured the process so kindly: David Acosta, Esther Acosta, Andrea Villaseñor, Debbie Walker, Lisa Kessenich, Dorita Lynch, Jenifer Villena, Cathy Kayne, Angel Alvarado, Elana Pisani, Karmel Bas, Petrina Gratton, Victoria Scribner, Brandy Jennings, Tashan Gavini, and Ramona Davoudpour, M.D. My thanks to each of you for your patience throughout this endeavor.

To those researchers and authors who granted me a moment of their busy schedules: Jill Stamm, Ph.D., Erica Komisar, LCSW, John Medina, Ph.D., Susannah Heschel, Robert Karen, Ph.D., Dmitri Christakis, Ph.D., Adrienne La France, Teresa Woodruff, Ph.D., Brett Finlay, Ph.D., Jay Belsky, Ph.D., and Susan Lynch, Ph.D.: Thank you, each of you, for enriching our understanding of the world we live in and thank you for granting me your personal attention and encouragement.

My nephew and office manager Casey Kessenich was ever helpful in tracking down articles and books and offering ideas from the very start. Thank you, Casey, for all that you have done!

For those who read portions of my book and made recommendations: Ben Bush, Barak Lurie, George Damascus, Robin Afrasiabi, Carlie Baiocchi, RNC-OB Natasha Beck, Psy.D., Harvey Karp, M.D., and Patricia Heaton, my sincere thanks for taking the time to make this book more readable and relevant.

To those whom I delegated many of my Africa mission responsibilities during this process: Cheryl Tormey, Dal Basile, and Patricia Peterson, special thanks for picking up the slack where I have fallen short.

Special thanks to my dear friend Harrison Sommer, my sagacious "sounding board" and Saturday-morning walking companion who has added helpful thoughts and comments from day one. Also to our lifelong friends Leon and Susan Hampton for their never-ending encouragement, to Dr. Gary and Eileen Brown for their ongoing emotional support, to Dennis and Barbara Metzler for their interest, to Gerri Coons who stood beside me as my nurse for over thirty years, to Dan Lieber, M.D., for his wise words, and finally, to my dear friend, thinker and inventor Darryl Massey for his enthusiasm and encouragement.

Also, special thanks to the pastors in my life who have been a source of both wisdom and insight: Pastor Harold Warner, whose integrity and vision I admire deeply; Pastor Bill Neil, who has heard my ramblings for longer than I want to admit; and Pastor Rob Scribner, who has been a source of inspiration for over thirty years.

I also want to thank my siblings who have quietly shared and supported this process with me: my brother, David Hamilton, and sisters, Katy Giannini and Debbie Grooms.

Special thanks to my beloved children: Joshua, Noel, Sarah, Peter, Emily, and Hannah Joy, all of whom have given me the ultimate full-color, firsthand experience in parenthood. I'm also thankful and appreciative of my seven lovely grandchildren: Nathan Hamilton, Levi Howard, Emery Jean, Hannah Jane, Bennett Robert, Louisa Anne, and John Julian who, by simply being *who they are* have enriched me and reminded me again of the blessings of parenthood.

My deepest honor and appreciation goes out to my father and mother, both of whom are now past. My parents guided me along a narrow path during the early stages of my life and provided a sure foundation from which I was able to build upon. Forever I will thank them for their great sacrifice in raising five children.

Finally, I want to thank my wife, Leslie, who is the *number one* joy of my life. I love her dearly. Since high school Leslie has been my ever-present confidante, a resource for practicality, and a never-ending treasure trove of good humor. She keeps my head out of the clouds and is my ultimate no-nonsense guide. Her unfailing belief that this project was worthy and her supporting prayers provided the soil for this project to grow.

Index

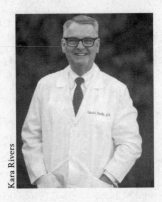

Kara Rivers

ROBERT C. HAMILTON, M.D., has more than three decades of experience as a pediatrician and is the owner
and founder of Pacific Ocean Pediatrics, established in
1996 in Santa Monica, California. Dr. Hamilton is also
the creator of the "Hamilton Hold," a method for soothing crying babies seen by over twenty-eight million people
in his instructional video on YouTube. In addition, Dr. Bob
runs the LA Marathon annually to support his medical
mission organization, which has been making annual
trips to both Africa and Central America for over twenty
years. He's also the proud father of six children and is
grandpa to eight more little ones. He lives in Santa Monica
with his high school sweetheart, Leslie, to whom he has
been married forty-five years.

SALLY COLLINGS is a writer and editor who has coau-
thored and collaborated on a string of bestselling and
award-winning titles, particularly in the field of well-
ness, relationships, and self-development. She lives in
the San Francisco Bay Area with her husband, two
daughters, and one calico cat.